The Healing
GARDEN

A *Practical*
GUIDE

FOR PHYSICAL
& EMOTIONAL

Well-being

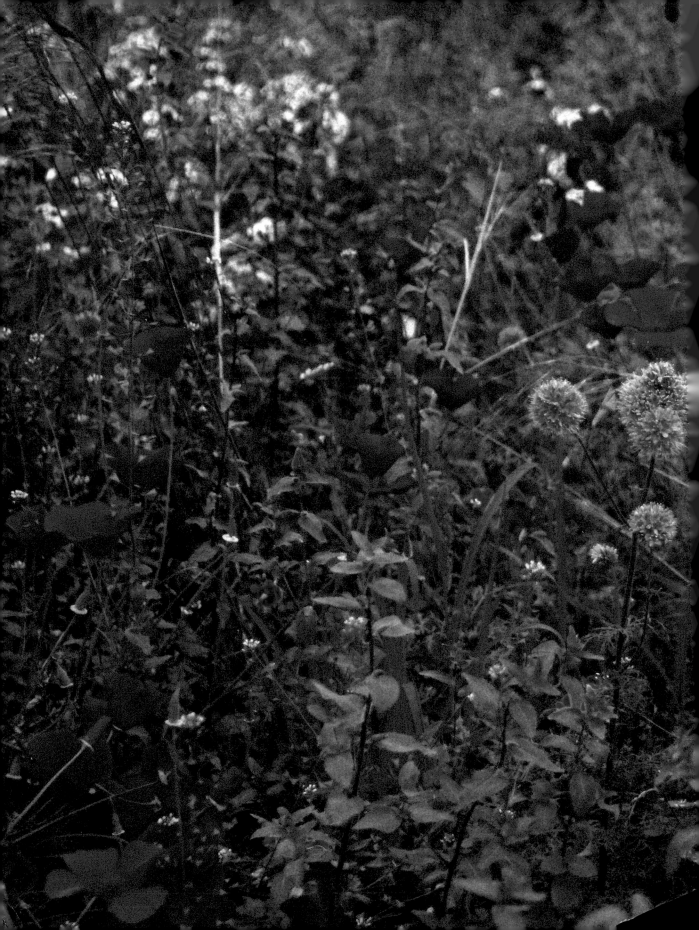

The Healing
GARDEN

A *Practical*
GUIDE
FOR PHYSICAL
& EMOTIONAL
Well-being

SUE MINTER

eden project books

TRANSWORLD PUBLISHERS
61–63 Uxbridge Road, London W5 5SA
a division of
The Random House Group Ltd

RANDOM HOUSE
AUSTRALIA (PTY) LTD
20 Alfred Street, Milsons Point, Sydney,
New South Wales 2061, Australia

RANDOM HOUSE
NEW ZEALAND LTD
18 Poland Road, Glenfield, Auckland 10,
New Zealand

RANDOM HOUSE
SOUTH AFRICA (PTY) LTD
Endulini, 5a Jubilee Road, Parktown 2193,
South Africa

First published 1993 by
Headline Book Publishing

First published in paperback 1994 by
Headline Book Publishing

Revised edition published 2005 by
Eden Project Books
a division of Transworld Publishers

Copyright © Sue Minter 2005
Design by Andrew Barron @ thextension
Picture Research: Vanessa Fletcher

Original concept by Geraldine Christy

A catalogue record for this book is
available from the British Library.
ISBN 1903 91941X

Typeset in Gill Sans and Baskerville

Printed in Germany

1 3 5 7 9 10 8 6 4 2

Papers used by Eden Project Books are
natural, recyclable products made from
wood grown in sustainable forests. The
manufacturing processes conform to the
environmental regulations of the country
of origin.

Note
Many of the plants mentioned in this
book are of medicinal use. However,
their description as such is no indication
of their safety and we strongly
recommend consultation with a qualified
medical practitioner before using them.

www.**books**at**transworld**.co.uk

Also by Sue Minter
The Apothecaries' Garden:
A History of Chelsea Physic Garden

TO PENNY WITH THANKS

CONTENTS

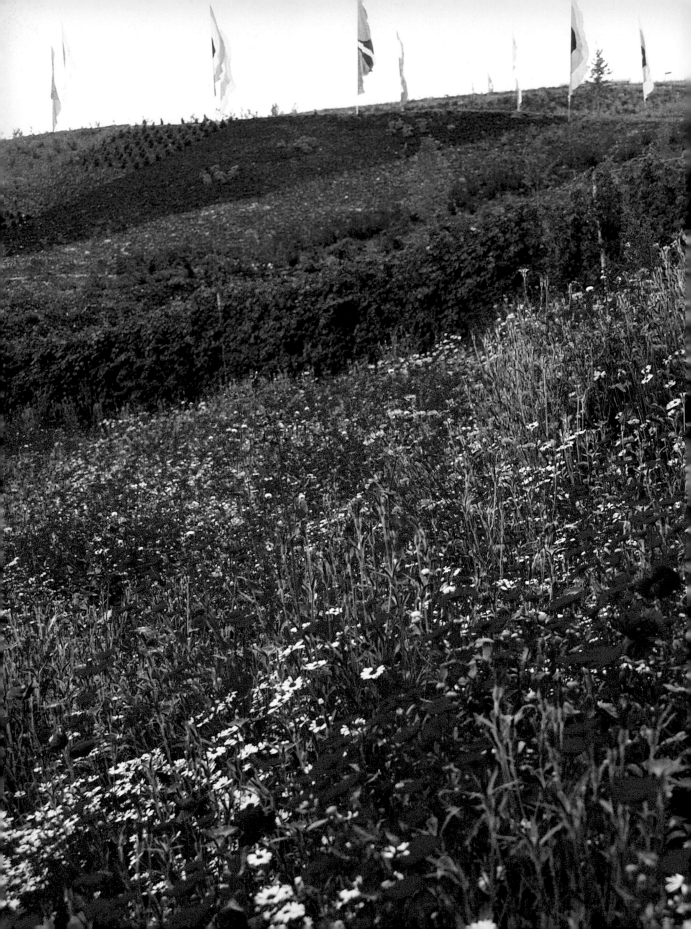

PREFACE

'ALL LIFE ON EARTH DEPENDS ON PLANTS', YET MANY OF US ONLY REALIZE THIS SIMPLE TRUTH THROUGH CONTACT WITH PLANTS IN OUR GARDENS. AND, FOR MANY, THE HEALING PROPERTIES OF PLANTS are hidden behind the way modern medicine presents them in the form of pills or ampoules.

In this book I want to show how plants are at the forefront of medicine and healthful nutrition and also to widen the definition of healing to include the way that gardens are used for recreation, self-expression and creative interplay with the natural world.

A 'WILDFLOWER MIX' SOWN AT THE EDEN PROJECT, CORNWALL, INCLUDES CORN DAISIES, CORN MARIGOLDS, FIELD POPPIES AND CORNFLOWERS.

Throughout the world our dependence on plants is a fact of everyday life to those who work with the soil and it is common to find rural societies with a highly developed sense of how to care for the environment and conserve it, in the belief that the land is 'not ours but borrowed from our children to come'. This unbroken thread of awareness and responsibility has been lost in more industrialized societies. Only 1.8 per cent of the British workforce now works in the agricultural sector. A recent survey by the (British) National Farmers' Union showed that only 35 per cent of the population had ever met a farmer, and in 2003 a survey co-ordinated for the Children's Society found that 80 per cent of children had been told off for playing outside.

This state of affairs is perhaps more extreme in Britain than in the rest of Europe because Britain was industrialized earlier. Far more smallholder agriculture still prevails in France, and Germany has a far more advanced ecological movement. Yet throughout Europe and the USA, as society continues to become more urbanized, so it becomes less familiar with the natural world and further removed from the sources of our food and medicines.

At the Chelsea Physic Garden in London, where I was Curator for ten years, visitors were amazed to see plants growing that are field-cropped for the production of pharmaceutical drugs like digoxin and morphine. Occasionally visitors whose lives had been saved by a drug from a plant became quite emotional when they saw it growing for the first time. (The sight of plants being cultivated for use in herbal and pharmaceutical medicine is more common in Eastern Europe.) I have anecdotal evidence that some visitors who distrusted pharmaceutical medicine felt better about the product once they knew it had plant origins. People seemed to welcome a link with a plant even if it was one step removed, as in the copying of a chemical template identified in a plant to produce a 'nature identical' product. Conversely, there seemed to be an instinctive distrust of anything synthesized, as if synthesis had become sinful. What a sea change from the day when Coco Chanel proudly launched her first 'totally synthetic' perfume in the 1930s. Yet we know that synthesis can sometimes save a species where extraction requires huge amounts of bulk material. Ephedra, for example, might have become endangered had ephedrine, which had been extracted from it and used in many patent medicines for catarrh, coughs and asthma, not been successfully synthesized.

This book makes connections between ideas about healing and how these link to plants. It takes a broad view; it does not seek to promote or endorse any particular system of healing (including the genetic technologies of the new millennium) but instead reviews the many ideas that humanity has produced about what illness is and how plants have been enlisted to help. It is also a practical book for gardeners, much of it based on my own experience, and gives advice on planning planting schemes, making garden features and using plants to create a garden that is healing for you as an individual.

The theme of our five senses – sight, hearing,

touch, taste and smell – recurs throughout the book. This is because it is our senses that reconnect us with the natural world and through which we can experience the garden as a healing place. The spiritual side of garden-making is also considered – how certain traditions of garden design have expressed the psychological needs of the societies that produced them, and how we can borrow from these in our own gardens for personal self-expression.

As I write I am aware of how the Eden Project has both grabbed the imagination of many millions of people and made them aware of plants as resources that must be marshalled sustainably if we are to go on living on this planet. The extent to which we rely on plant material is brought home to the visitors in an animatronic (puppet) display called 'Plant Takeaway'. It shows a family who have everything made from plants stripped out of their lives; they lose all their clothes, food

and furniture and end up totally naked, dying from lack of oxygen. The search for the family's lost plant products forms the basis of one of the trails around the biomes. The Project's own landscape, which was once an industrial scar and is now 'healed', is a pointer to the potential of plants to create a healing space. Perhaps the renewed recognition of the value of the world of plants and what it can offer us augurs well for an age which is struggling to contain the many pressures on our environment and is desperate for a sense of optimism. Let us hope so.

Sue Minter
April 2004

PLANT HARDINESS ZONES

The zone given for each plant represents its tolerance of winter cold in Western Europe; in climates with hotter and/or drier summers, as in the United States, Australia and New Zealand, some plants will survive colder temperatures. The chart opposite indicates the average annual minimum temperature of each zone. Zoning can only give a rough guideline. Plant hardiness depends on a great many factors, such as the depth of a plant's roots, the rate at which the temperature falls, the duration of cold weather and wind force. Also, within any one zone, particular regions may be endowed with more or less favourable conditions.

Celsius	Zone	Fahrenheit
Below −45	1	Below −50
−45 to −40	2	−50 to −40
−40 to −34	3	−40 to −30
−34 to −29	4	−30 to −20
−29 to −23	5	−20 to −10
−23 to −18	6	−10 to 0
−18 to −12	7	0 to 10
−12 to −7	8	10 to 20
−7 to −1	9	20 to 30
−1 to 4	10	30 to 40

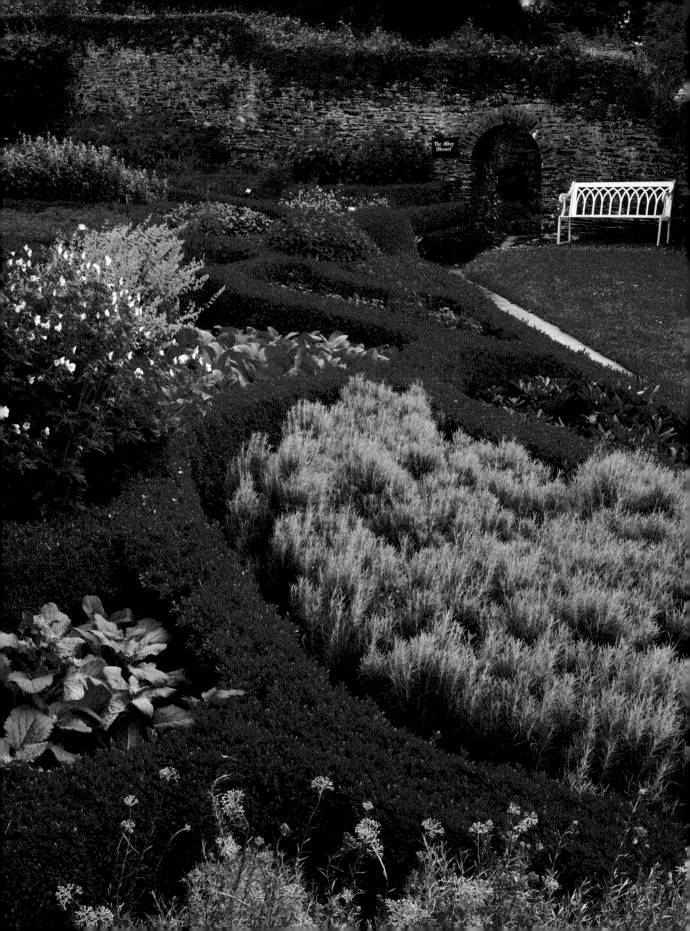

The Abbey
(House)

THE HEALING

ARTS

'THERE IS NO ILLNESS BUT THERE IS A PLANT TO CURE IT.' THIS BELIEF WAS AT THE ROOT OF ALL MEDICINE FROM ANCIENT EGYPT TO RENAISSANCE EUROPE. THE ENTIRE COUNTRYSIDE WAS NATURE'S pharmacy, and healers identified their plants by descriptions and illustrations in medicinal handbooks known as herbals. Monastery, guild and university 'physic' gardens were established so that 'physicians' could study and use the principal healing plants collected together in one place. From these gardens developed the modern botanic garden.

Today many societies all over the world still understand the importance of plants in medicine and either grow them for their own use, collect them from the wild or trade in them in medicinal plant markets. As the consumer of a capsule, tablet or ampoule you are unlikely to be aware of how many of these medicines have been derived from plants, or how they are produced. How much better it would be if we could choose to buy products on the basis of knowledge about the issues involved in their production.

A RECREATED PHYSIC GARDEN OF HEALING PLANTS AT
BUCKLAND ABBEY IN DEVON. MONASTERIES WERE CENTRES OF HEALING IN
THE WEST THROUGHOUT THE MIDDLE AGES.

THE ANCIENT ART OF HEALING

Over the centuries answers to the question 'What is healing?' have ranged from the purely practical to complex philosophies based on the relation of human beings to the natural, religious or supernatural world order. Cultures have differed in their systems of healing, although many have stressed the importance of maintaining some sort of balance within the individual. Almost without exception, however, all cultures have used plants in some way to cure ailments and prevent illness.

The earliest roots of medicine in the cultures that developed from the Middle Eastern cradles of civilization lay in Mesopotamia where, from 4000 to 1500 BC, disease was thought to be inflicted by the gods and treatment was by exorcism. From about 2000 BC, however, this supernatural approach was gradually superseded by an attention to symptoms, which were treated both by propitiating charms and by plant-based medicines.

The Egyptians also maintained parallel beliefs in both the supernatural and in the natural causes of illness. They developed a widespread cultivation of drug plants – they were the first to use senna and castor oil as laxatives, and in Roman times became the chief exporters of opium. Physicians like Imhotep of the Third Dynasty were famous for prescribing drugs in association with religious rituals. The physicians' patron was Thoth, the scribe god of knowledge, and they established a renowned medical library in the city of Alexandria.

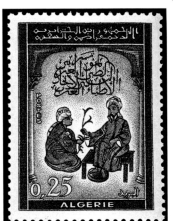

AN ALGERIAN POSTAGE STAMP CELEBRATES THE TRANSMISSION OF KNOWLEDGE ABOUT MEDICINAL PLANTS FROM HEALER TO APPRENTICE.

In Greece, Aristotle (384–322 BC) played down the importance of the supernatural and developed a 'logical' view of the human body being composed of four 'humours', an idea that was first proposed by the many authors of the *Hippocratic Corpus* of the fifth century BC. According to him, these humours, or liquids (blood, phlegm, yellow bile and black bile), should be held in balance and affected the body as a microcosm of the world order just as earth, air, fire and water affected the world itself, the macrocosm. It is easy to see how these concepts later became translated into medieval and Renaissance views on alchemy and astrology. Paralleling Aristotle's philosophical ideas on the maintenance of health through balancing the humours was the more practical work of Theophrastus (371–287 BC), who described over 550 species of plants and their medicinal uses in maintaining this balance. The Greeks also dedicated temples to the healer god

Asclepius as centres of healing, and at the sanctuary of Epidaurus votive offerings modelled on the part of the body cured would be displayed.

The Romans based their medical systems on those of the Greeks. Their most notable source was *De Materia Medica,* by Dioscorides (AD 40–90), an army doctor from Asia Minor. Dioscorides discussed the medicinal use of over 600 plants, including belladonna and opium, and illustrated from nature the plants he used; and his book became standard in Europe well into medieval times. It was used by the Greek physician Galen (AD 129–199), who refined Aristotle's ideas for his practice in Rome and developed a coherent system of physiology and anatomy.

The traditions of the Greeks and Romans survived the Dark Ages that followed the fall of Rome largely through their use in the Islamic world. In Persia, the physician Ibn Sina (AD 980–1037), known in the West as Avicenna, preserved the work of Galen and Aristotle and considerably advanced drug therapy with his complex blending of ingredients, most of which remained plant-based.

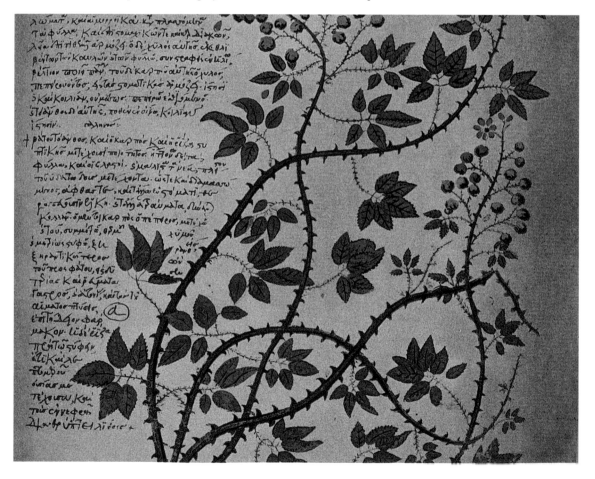

HERBALS WERE LIKE FIELD GUIDES TO ASSIST IN THE ACCURATE IDENTIFICATION OF MEDICINAL PLANTS. ANNOTATIONS LISTED THE PLANTS' THERAPEUTIC USE.

THE BEGINNINGS OF WESTERN MEDICINE

After the fall of Rome the main medical theories in the West continued to follow the principle of the Aristotelian humours, and the work of Dioscorides provided a source of reference for plant-based drugs. The treatment of illnesses consisted of restoring the 'balance of the humours' by purging, by various forms of blood-letting (bleeding and cupping) and by the medicinal use of herbs. Diagnosis was made by studying the patient's urine. In the Christian tradition offerings were often made to saints to invoke their protection against disease, while fragrant oils from plants were used to fumigate rooms to ward off the plague (see page 132).

During the Renaissance enormous conceptual changes radically affected medical thought. On the one hand the idea of the body as a machine was developing, clearly illustrated in the drawings of Leonardo da Vinci (1452–1519) and later in the writings of the French philosopher and mathematician René Descartes (1596–1650). This stimulated medical knowledge by encouraging dissection (the first anatomy theatre was opened in Padua in 1594), which in turn led to a development in medical instruments. On the other hand there was a growing interest in astrology based on the Hippocratic and Aristotelian view of humans as microcosms that are affected by the analogous macrocosm of the heavens. Alchemy was also rooted in the microcosm and macrocosm theory. The Swiss physician Paracelsus (1493–1541) believed that the body functioned as a model of the chemical reactions of

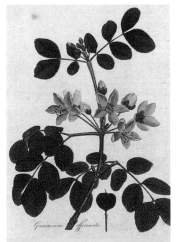

GUAIACUM OFFICINALE WAS INTRODUCED TO EUROPE BY THE SPANISH AND USED FOR THAT NEW WORLD DISEASE – SYPHILIS.

the entire universe. Since illnesses were due to chemical imbalance, they could be cured by treating the patient with chemicals. These included mercury and antimony, now known to be highly toxic. The most widely known medical astrologer, famed for his book *The English Physician* (1653), was the herbalist Nicholas Culpeper, who promoted the use of plants for medicinal use in the English language.

The real development in plant-based medicine, however, came not from new theories about illness but from travel. Following Columbus's so-called discovery of the Americas in 1492 came the introduction in Europe of aloes (used as a purgative), quinine (for fever), guaiacum (for syphilis), coca and tobacco (originally thought to be of high medicinal value, perhaps because of its use by native Americans). With the successful navigation of the route to the Far East in 1498 came rhubarb root from India (used as a purgative), senna from Africa and camphor (used as an insect-repellent and rubrifacient) from Japan. These and many other plants, such as ipecacuanha (an American treatment for dysentery), were cultivated in the botanic gardens of Renaissance Europe.

The physic garden tradition

The earliest moves towards the concept of a botanic garden began at least 1000 years BC in the ancient Egyptian temple gardens, where known medicinal plants were grown. The Greeks developed botany as a philosophical study before the time of Christ and in China the reigning emperors became some of the earliest people to collect plants.

In Europe, however, it was in monasteries from the sixth century AD onwards that medicinal gardens became standard, and were sited next to the infirmary. Botany was firmly wedded to medicine and, with the foundation of the early universities during the Renaissance, the professors of the one discipline were usually also the professors of the other. Still paying respect to the old ideas of Paracelsus and Dioscorides, plants were seen as being present on earth for their healing benefit, known or potential. They were grown in 'physick' gardens to serve the physicians' requirements for existing or newly introduced raw materials in the healing arts and to teach medical students to distinguish between what would cure and what would kill their patients. There was no concept of botany as a systematic discipline in its own right; that idea,

which is fundamental to the idea of a modern botanic garden, developed later in the eighteenth and nineteenth centuries with the introduction of new taxonomic (plant naming) systems.

All the early physic gardens, which were generally walled against wind and marauders and laid out formally, were products of the Italian Renaissance. The first was established in Pisa in 1543; the second in 1543 in Padua (now a World Heritage Site); another in Florence in 1550. Other countries followed suit with gardens at Leipzig (1580), Heidelburg (1593), Paris (1635) and Uppsala (1665), and also at Leiden (1587), where there is a charming re-creation of the original *hortus clusianus*. In Britain the first university garden was at Oxford; founded in 1621, it retained its original name of the Oxford Physic Garden until 1840, by when medical botany was in disfavour compared to the rising independent science of systematic and observational botany. Similarly, Edinburgh's Physic Garden, founded in 1656, is now its Botanic Garden; the Chelsea Physic Garden in London, which was founded in 1673 for training the apprentices of the Society of Apothecaries, is the only ancient British physic garden to have kept its title.

There is now a move to create or restore physic gardens, particularly in the USA under the aegis of the American Herb Society, for example at Morristown, New Jersey, and Yellow Springs, Pennsylvania. In Britain modern physic gardens with an educational and display purpose can be seen at Petersfield in Hampshire and at Hitchin in Hertfordshire.

MEDICAL SYSTEMS FROM AROUND THE WORLD

There are many traditions of healing from around the world that run parallel to the type of medicine practised in the West. One of the most ancient is the Indian Ayurvedic system, which is common at a community level in India, particularly southern India. In Africa, the Americas, and in Australia and New Zealand, the indigenous peoples have their own medicinal practices using plants. Their ideas about healing are deeply rooted in their culture and traditions. Some have used plant drugs that have subsequently been adopted by Western medicine and double-blind tested for efficacy.

Indian Ayurvedic healing

Of all the ancient systems of medicine the one closest to the Aristotelian tradition of humours is Indian. 'Ayurveda' in Sanskrit means 'the science of life' or 'the science of [living to a ripe] age' and was dominant in the Indian subcontinent from 1500 BC until the tenth century AD. Ayurvedic doctors believe that there are seven 'dhatus' or elements (food juices, flesh, blood, fat, bones, marrow and semen) in the body and three 'tridosa' or humours (wind, bile and phlegm). In the body of a healthy person there is a good balance between the dhatus and the tridosa which may be affected by the constitution that you inherit. The principal Ayurvedic texts, the *Caralea Samhita* and the *Susruta Samhita*, date from 200 BC to AD 200 and include over 700 useful herbs classified by their action on the dhatus and tridosa, or by their effects on the patient. The tra-

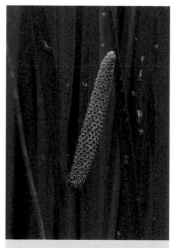

ACORUS CALAMUS IS USED IN AYURVEDIC MEDICINE, THOUGH BANNED IN THE USA. IT IS ENDANGERED IN THE WILD.

dition also stresses the need to collect the plant drugs in the right way, at the right season and from the right soil. The purity of the doctor and the way the drugs are stored are considered important, as is the patient's diet.

Today, Ayurveda is widely used in India as a matter of cultural preference and an inexpensive alternative to expensive Western drugs. It is also practised in Sri Lanka, where many people believe that the humoral balance can be disturbed by demons that need to be exorcized. In Britain, Ayurveda is used by Asian communities and there is now an Ayurvedic Company of Great Britain working in association with a pharmacy in Coimbatore, southern India, that manages two therapy centres. Much of the therapy consists of the use of herbal oils in massage and of diet control; it is claimed to be particularly effective in treating rheumatic diseases. Ayurveda has been

THE POURING OF OILS, MEDICATED WITH PLANTS FOR ABSORPTION INTO THE SCALP (OPPOSITE), IS CALLED 'SIROVASTHI' IN AYURVEDIC PRACTICE IN INDIA.

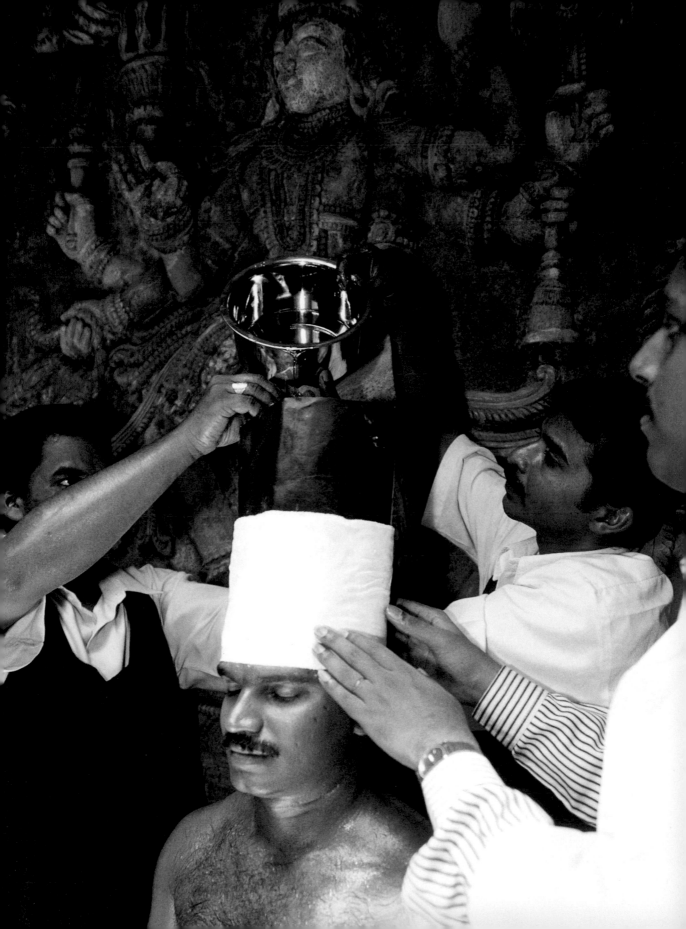

criticized, however, for the inclusion of heavy metals in its medicines, which are now known to be toxic, especially to children.

Acupuncture and the Chinese *Pharmacopoeia*

The Chinese, in common with the ancient Greeks and Romans, have a history of linking health with divine influence. They also have a very solid tradition of plant-based medicine dating from the first and second centuries BC, when the delightfully named *Pharmacopoeia of the Heavenly Husbandman* listed over 300 drugs. From the sixth century BC physicians had used *The Yellow Emperor's Manual of Corporeal Medicine,* and by the time of the Ming Dynasty (1368–1644) their art had developed to a high point. Thereafter, medical practice became divided into the philosophical and the practical, the latter becoming increasingly superstitious until the arrival of communism. Much of the treatment was nevertheless plant-based, perhaps influenced by the Taoist tradition of venerating nature by observation.

In parallel with the use of drugs was an interest in massage, gymnastics and acupuncture. Acupuncture was first used in about 500 BC and, although temporarily banned in 1822, is still used extensively in modern China's system of devolved health care; it is also becoming increasingly widely used in complementary medicine in the West. Acupuncture involves the insertion of fine needles into the body at certain defined points that are said to be joined by invisible meridians (the twelve Ching) and two auxiliary tracts (Ho). Energy (Chi) passes along these tracts and the treatment by needles aims to restore the flow if it has become blocked or disrupted. Acupuncturists use plants as well, particularly where disease is severe, by burning small cones of powdered *Artemisia vulgaris* leaves (moxa) for precise lengths of time at specific points around the body. This technique is called moxibustion and was also used in the Japanese system of traditional medicine (Kampo), at least until the adoption of Western medical practice in Japan after the 1870s.

Today, Traditional Chinese Medicine (TCM) is a sizeable and expanding presence in Britain through retail pharmacies. These serve the Chinese immigrant population and are attracting increasing interest from the non-Chinese community. There has been a programme at the Royal Botanic Gardens, Kew, near London, assisting the Chinese community in regulating the quality control of their imports of plants and preventing adulteration and poisonings.

African traditions

Many African cultures traditionally believe that disease is caused by the malevolence of witches, sorcerers or evil ancestors, and medicinal healers are therefore a spiritual focus in the community. It is believed that disease can be avoided by observing taboos, wearing amulets, giving offerings to beneficent ancestors or ritual dancing. This spiritual approach is backed up by the use of the local flora by herbalists, although the herbal drugs are generally thought to be more effective when used in conjunction with charms and chants. Local markets are often rich in medicinal plants that are either cultivated or plucked from the wild. South

Africa has a particularly strong herbal tradition working alongside Western medicine.

North American medicine

North American Indians have developed very distinct theories as to the spiritual causes of disease. Illness is thought to result from 'soul loss' where the soul has been kidnapped by a ghost or an enemy, by the intrusion of an object into the body through sorcery or by the breaking of a strongly held taboo.

The practice of the medicine man relates to the plant world in several ways. Some tribes believe that spirits inspire the healer to know which curative plants to use, others that a plant is protected by the spirit that has endowed it with medicinal properties. Offerings are often left to these spirits when the drug plant is picked. Healing is indicated by the return of the soul or by the medicine man claiming to produce the 'extracted object'. Massage and ritual 'sweat baths' are also used in the healing process.

Drugs of the ancient American civilizations

In Mexico the ancient civilizations of the Mayas and the Aztecs had a strong social hierarchy; astrologer-diviners served the medicinal needs of the nobility, and herbalists served those of the majority of the people. The Incas of Peru had similar beliefs to those of the North American Indian tribes and used plants that are well known today, including curare for digestive diseases. Cocaine was used ritualistically by healers; and quinine was known to be useful against fever long before it was discovered by the Jesuits, although the explana-

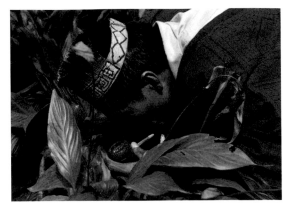

tion of its action – that the disease-causing spirit could not bear its bitterness – was peculiarly Indian. Tobacco was a common drug used throughout the Americas; it was deified in Mexico, used as a sedative in Peru and played a part in much of North American Indian life as a social ritual.

Aboriginal and Maori traditions

The Australian Aborigines traditionally believe that illness is caused by sorcery, particularly by the insertion of objects such as needles or slivers of bone. The tribal elders, in contact with their Dreaming, would claim to extract the objects. Medicinal plants were, and still are, used. Anyone who has ever had a pre-med injection before an anaesthetic for surgery will have received a drug called hyoscine, which is commercially cropped from *Duboisia myoporoides*, a medicinal plant well known to the Aborigines.

Maori culture stressed the avoidance of disease by appeasing their ancestors, observing taboos and deflecting the wrath of the gods. As with most invaded cultures, the Maori began to contract the diseases the settlers brought with them.

A PERUVIAN SHAMAN PARTICIPATES IN THE CEREMONY OF 'AYAHUASCA', USING HALLUCINOGENS IN A VINE TO INSPIRE DIAGNOSTIC VISIONS.

HERBALISM

Herbalism has its origins in an age-old basic belief that plants exist to provide remedies for the body's ills; it is fundamentally different to homoeopathy, which is an eighteenth-century tradition based on much non-plant material.

In medieval times, and up until the seventeenth century, the knowledge and lore of herbs was written down in herbals. These books were sometimes illustrated with woodcuts, often done by monks who simply copied the illustrations of plants from their forebears until they became either crudely diagrammatic or totally fanciful. With the Renaissance, however, came an interest in observing and drawing real plants from nature, and some of the herbals, those of Otto Brunfels (*Herbarum Vivae Eicones*, 1541–2) and Leonard Fuchs (*De Historia Stirpium*, 1542) for example, are absolute gems of plant portraiture. In England the most famous herbals were those of John Gerard in 1633 and Nicholas Culpeper in 1653.

Nevertheless, this written tradition should not blind us to the fact that a lot of knowledge was (and still is) passed on from generation to generation by word of mouth. Generally, especially in medieval times, women were the 'herb gatherers' and it was the lower classes of society who relied on their wares. Educated and wealthier people preferred to be treated with the mineral-based drugs of physicians. By the eighteenth century

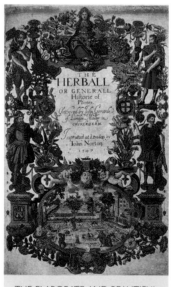

THE ELABORATE AND BEAUTIFUL FRONTISPIECE TO JOHN GERARD'S *HERBALL* OF 1633.

herbalism had lost its popularity, although it remained in practice in the poor, rural areas of Europe and also in colonial America.

In order to help restore confidence in herbalism, the National Association of Medical Herbalists was formed in Britain in 1864; it offered training and qualifications and established recognized codes of practice. This organization still exists (as the National Institute of Medical Herbalists), the oldest professional body of its kind, and herbalists who are registered with it carry the initials MNIMH after their names.

About 85 per cent of the global population still relies on herbalism for its basic health care, and many use herbal remedies in preference to pharmaceutical medicines. (Modern herbalism uses a rich variety of vegetable matter, not just the culinary and aromatic 'herbs' with which we are familiar in the kitchen.) This is not to say that all herbal remedies are proven, however, nor to say that all 'natural' plant remedies are gentle and harmless; after all, some of the most deadly poisons come from plants.

Sometimes herbal remedies have been taken

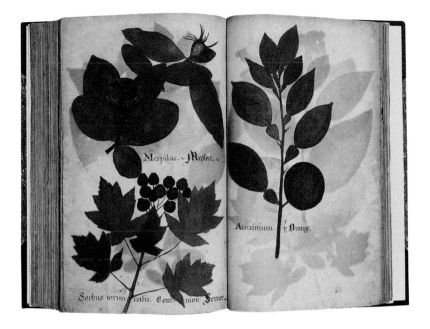

Mespilus. Medlar.

Aurantium. y Orange.

Sorbus torminalis. Common Service.

up by orthodox Western medicine, tested and been proved effective according to double-blind testing. An example is ginger, which contains a substance that counters motion sickness more effectively than synthetic drugs.

There remains, however, a basic conflict between the theory that underlies herbalism and that which supports orthodox medicine. The herbalist believes that the healing properties of the whole plant work together and rejects the isolation of a chemical principle from it. Orthodox medicine dismisses this as a theory with no firm scientific evidence, and pharmaceutical companies continue to screen plants for active chemical principles, isolating them and often synthesizing them chemically for prescription as drugs. A biochemist once suggested to me that these opposing views could be reconciled by the notion that chemicals within the plant act together (synergis-

tically) to create a healing effect. The main point, though, is that the herbalist trusts the effect of the plant itself rather than chemistry. This approach appeals to many people because they have experienced side effects from synthetic drugs or because they wish to return to a type of healing that seems closer to nature. It is probably these factors (as well as a general movement towards self-treatment) that have led to the huge interest in herbal medicine in the West in recent times.

Herbalists generally prescribe medicines in the form of alcohol-based tinctures, and only after a long discussion with the patient to ascertain his or her emotional and psychological state and any other circumstantial factors that may affect the holistic diagnosis. In this regard herbalists are similar to homoeopaths (see page 24) in their holistic consultation procedure.

THE UNIQUE *ICONES* OF JOSEPH MILLER (1772) AT THE CHELSEA PHYSIC GARDEN
IS A NATURE-PRINTED NOTEBOOK OF MEDICINAL PLANTS.

HOMOEOPATHY

Homoeopathy is a system of healing in which like is treated with like, a principle known to the Greek physician Hippocrates in the fifth century BC but not developed until the eighteenth century in Germany. Its chief proponent was Dr Samuel Hahnemann (1755–99), who was concerned by the harsh medical approaches of the time in which blood-letting and the use of arsenic were common. He coined the name 'homoeopathy' for the new method from the Greek *homoios* meaning 'like' to differentiate it from conventional or 'allopathic' medicine (from the Greek *allos* meaning 'other'), which used drugs to fight against disease.

At the heart of the system is a different approach to the meaning of medical symptoms. Orthodox medicine maintains that these result from the disease and need to be suppressed, or counteracted. Homoeopaths claim that the symptoms express the body's attempt to heal itself and, indeed, may need to be encouraged.

In homoeopathy, substances that produce the same symptoms as those of the disease itself are used as cures. Not all of these are plant-based – almost half of the major cures derive from vegetable matter, the rest being brought about by mineral salts, or animal or other biological materials. Hahnemann is said to have been led to his ideas by observing how a plant (cinchona bark) produced fever in a healthy person, yet cured malaria.

Homoeopathy qualifies as a 'holistic' therapy because it concentrates on all the facets of a person – spiritual, mental and emotional as well as physical. Each of these facets can affect the progress of a disease and each needs to be assessed before an appropriate treatment can be selected. New patients often find it strange to have their appearance, reactions, beliefs and fears assessed as well as their symptoms. The aim is to restore health by restoring balance so that the body can heal itself, thus healing the person and not treating the disease. In a complex or prolonged cure, homoeopaths believe that the symptoms of a disease may worsen before they are relieved and that previous symptoms may resurface before disappearing. Symptoms can also 'move' about the body in the process of healing, from internal organs to more superficial sites.

Probably the most controversial side of homoeopathy is the belief that the remedies are made more potent by extreme dilution, while also being made safer. Allopathic doctors often say that the dilution is so great that scarcely a molecule of the original substance can remain. Homoeopaths respond that they do not know how their system works, but that they see that it does.

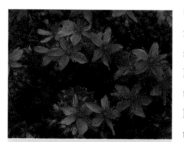

HYPERICUM IS USED IN BOTH HERBAL MEDICINE AND HOMOEOPATHY AS A WOUND HERB.

ACONITUM NAPELLUS, COMMONLY KNOWN AS MONKSHOOD (OPPOSITE), IS EXTREMELY TOXIC BUT USED IN HOMOEOPATHY IN MINUTE DOSES.

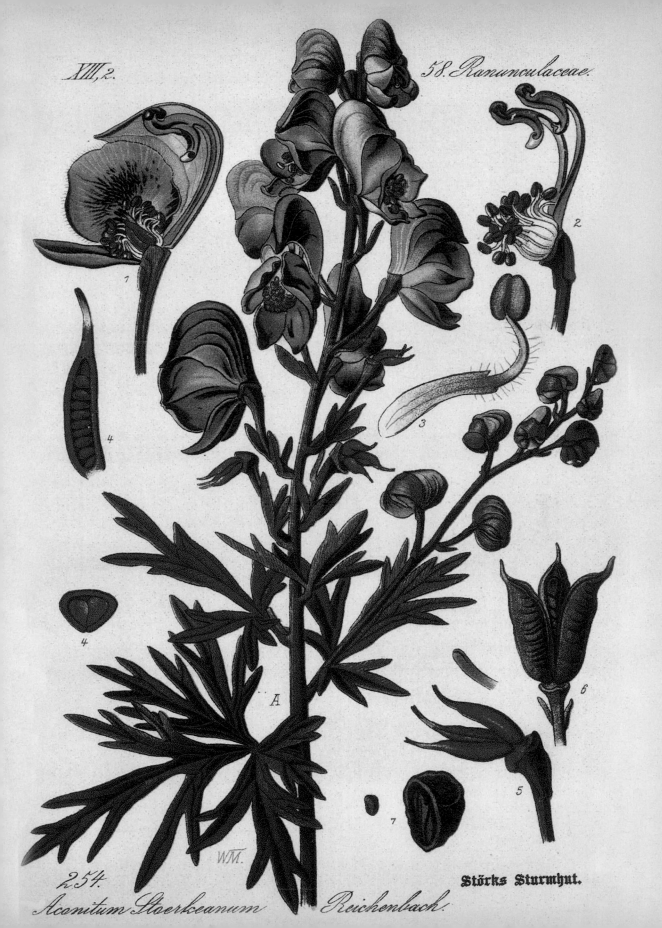

Störks Sturmhut.

Aconitum Stoerkeanum Reichenbach.

PLANT REMEDIES USED IN HOMOEOPATHY

Name: Botanical; Common; Homoeopathic	Physical symptoms	Emotional state
Aconitum napellus; Aconite; Aconite	Sudden chill, dry cough, sore throat following chill, fever with thirst, intense pain, motion sickness, insomnia.	Bereavement or grief, anxiety, fear, restlessness, panic attacks.
Actaea spicata; Baneberry; Actaea	Headache, neuralgia, muscle strain, rheumatic stiffness in upper body.	Depression, confusion.
Arnica montana; Arnica; Arnica	Bruises, sprains, muscle strain, gout, rheumatism.	Overtiredness, sensitivity to being touched.
Atropa belladonna; Deadly Nightshade; Belladonna	Swelling of joints, neuralgia, earache, throbbing headache, dry cough, motion sickness and vertigo, acne, cystitis, colic, insomnia.	Lively cheerful disposition.
Bryonia alba; White Bryony; Bryonia	Chesty colds, pleurisy, dry cough, dry lips, thirst, colic, arthritis.	Irritable.
†*Cephaelis (Psychotria) ipecacuanha*; Ipecacuanha; Ipecacuanha	Nausea, sickness, bronchitis, breathlessness.	–
Drosera rotundifolia; Sundew; Drosera	Coughs, sickness, laryngitis, vertigo.	–
Euphrasia officinialis; Eyebright; Euphrasia	Streaming colds, conjunctivitis, sensitivity to strong light, hayfever, eye strain.	–
†*Gelsemium sempervirens*; Carolina Jasmine; Gelsemium	Influenza and its symptoms, absence of thirst with fever, delirium, difficulty in swallowing.	Nervous excitability, worry, phobic personality.
Hamamelis virginiana; Witch Hazel; Hamamelis	Varicose veins, nosebleeds, bleeding piles, tired and sore limbs, chilblains.	–
Hypericum perforatum; St John's Wort; Hypericum	Painful wounds, injuries from falls, injured fingers and toes, piles, insect bites.	–
Lycopodium clavatum; Club Moss; Lycopodium	Hunger cravings, especially for sweet things, stomach irritability, cystitis, menstrual problems, premature baldness and greying.	Irritability, fear of failure, intenseness and insecurity, unsociability.
Pulsatilla pratensis ssp. *nigricans*; Pulsatilla; Pulsatilla	Catarrh, hayfever, styes, period pain or irregularity, premenstrual tension, cystitis, acne, tinnitus, arthritis, dry mouth.	Affectionate, responsive, weepy.
Ruta graveolens; Rue; Ruta graveolens	Fractures, sprains, dislocations, rheumatism, arthritis, eye strain, nettle rash.	–

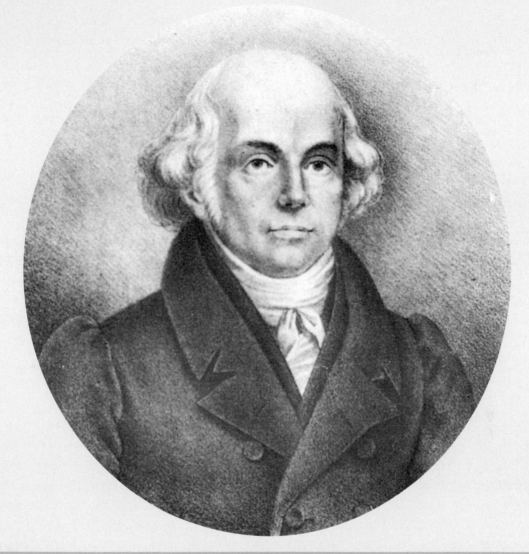

• †*Strychnos nux-vomica*; Nux Vomica; Nux Vomica	Nervous indigestion, liverishness, constipation, piles, premenstrual tension.	Impatience, irritability, anxiousness.
*Thuja occidentalis; White Cedar; Thuja	Warts, styes, frequent urination, headaches.	Strong, stubborn and opinionated.
• *Toxicodendron radicans*; Poison Ivy; *Rhus toxicodendron*	Strains and sprains, sciatica, rheumatism, lumbago, arthritis, shingles, thirst, cold sores.	Restlessness.

* Easily cultivated in gardens with temperate climates   † Tropical species   • Not recommended for cultivation

SAMUEL HAHNEMANN WAS THE ORIGINATOR OF THE THEORY OF HOMOEOPATHY –
THAT 'LIKE CURES LIKE' AND DOES SO VIA MINUTE DOSAGES.

AROMATHERAPY

Aromatherapy is curative treatment based on the use of essential oils derived from plants. Its history is pre-Christian and the principal ancient cultures that practised it were Chinese, Egyptian, Greek and Roman, all of which used aromatic oils, although the oils were probably infused rather than distilled.

The 'royal gifts' of frankincense and myrrh given to the child Christ attest the importance of plant aromas in religious practices. *Boswellia carteri* and *Commiphora myrrha* are both resinous trees of the semi-desert areas of North East Africa and have a long tradition of use. Incense was used in Egypt on state occasions and the pyramids have yielded the remains of ointments and oils. From Egypt the use of aromatic plants passed to the Greeks, and thence to the Arabs, who first invented the process of distilling essential oils from the resinous woody species of their homelands. Some sources have credited the discovery to the Persian physician Ibn Sina (see page 15) in the eleventh century. The perfumes of Arabia were as sought after by the Crusaders as were the 'spices of the Orient' by the seventeenth-century explorers of the Far East. For the southern Europeans the equivalent of the resinous trees of Arabia were their native aromatics, such as rosemary, lavender and thyme, and oils from these plants were sold to the general population by druggists and apothecaries.

The popularity of aromatherapy today derives from work done almost entirely by the Frenchmen René-Maurice Gattefossé and Jean Valnet, and some of the best-known manufacturers of aromatherapy oils are French.

Aromatherapy is mostly empirically based – that is, the effects of oils are determined by observation; however, some aromatherapists subscribe to complex theories concerning the way the oils are absorbed and heal via meridians in the body.

Essential oils are absorbed through the skin and by inhalation. The most popular uses are in massage (where the oil or blend of oils is mixed with a carrier oil), in bathing, and by creams, lotions and compresses. Anyone using oils regularly should consult a trained aromatherapist, as some oils can be toxic. Many of these oils are expensive because a large quantity of plant material is necessary to produce a small drop of oil. Some are also the products of tropical species, particularly the exotic and supposedly aphrodisiac ones, and so cannot be grown outdoors in a temperate climate. Many others, however, are derived from plants that can be grown in an 'aromatherapy garden' for your own interest and delight, though you are unlikely to be able to grow enough for commercial cropping.

A BOTANICAL PAINTING OF *BOSWELLIA CARTERI*. FRANKINCENSE IS THE RESIN COLLECTED FROM THIS SHRUB.

A TABLE OF AROMATHERAPY OILS

The following table lists aromatherapy oils and the botanical name of the species from which they are obtained. All, except the tropical species, can be grown outside but it is best to take those that are marked with an asterisk (first column) into a cool greenhouse over winter. In general, aromatherapy oils are safe providing they are applied to the skin in a carrier oil and not neat. However, do heed the warnings given.

Common name	Botanical name	Warning	Reputed effect
TEMPERATE OILS			
Basil*	Ocimum basilicum	● ■	Uplifting, stimulating.
Bergamot	Citrus bergamia	■ ✳	Refreshing, analgesic, anti-depressant, antiseptic.
Camomile	Chamaemelum nobile		Refreshing, analgesic, anti-depressant, febrifuge.
Clary Sage	Salvia sclarea	●	Warming, aphrodisiac, anti-depressant, calming.
Cypress	Cupressus sempervirens		Refreshing, deodorant.
Eucalyptus	Eucalyptus globulus		Warming, antiseptic, expectorant, febrifuge.
Geranium*	Pelargonium odoratissimum		Refreshing, relaxing, anti-depressant.
Juniper	Juniperus communis	●	Refreshing, stimulating, detoxifying.
Lavender	Lavandula angustifolia		Refreshing, relaxing, analgesic, antiseptic.
Lemon*	Citrus limonum	■ ✳	Refreshing, stimulating.
Lemon Verbena*	Aloysia triphylla	■ ✳	Antiseptic, insect-repellent.
Marjoram	Origanum majorana	●	Warming, analgesic, relaxing.
Melissa	Melissa officinalis	■	Uplifting, anti-depressant, febrifuge.
Neroli*	Citrus aurantium	■ ✳	Very relaxing, anti-depressant, aphrodisiac.
Peppermint	Mentha piperita	● ■	Cooling, stimulating.
Petigrain*	Citrus bigaradia	✳ ■	Refreshing, anti-depressant.
Pine Needle	Pinus sylvestris		Refreshing, antiseptic.
Rose	Rosa centifolia/damascena	●	Relaxing, soothing, anti-depressant, aphrodisiac.
Rosemary	Rosmarinus officinalis	● ▲	Invigorating, analgesic, antiseptic.
Tarragon*	Artemisia dracunculus		Warming.
Thyme	Thymus vulgaris	■ ▲	Antiseptic.
TROPICAL OILS			
Benzoin	Styrax benzoin		Warming, relaxing, expectorant, wound-healing.
Black Pepper	Piper nigrum		Stimulating, warming.
Frankincense	Boswellia carteri		Relaxing, reviving, astringent.
Ginger	Zingiber officinale		Warming, digestive.
Jasmine	Jasminum grandiflorum		Soothing, anti-depressant, aphrodisiac.
Lemongrass	Cymbopogon citratus	■	Tonic, refreshing.
Myrrh	Commiphora myrrha	●	Cooling, tonic, anti-inflammatory, fungicidal.
Patchouli	Pogostemon patchouli		Relaxing.
Tea Tree	Melaleuca alternifolia	■	Antiseptic, antiviral, febrifuge, tonic.
Ylang-Ylang	Cananga odorata		Relaxing, aphrodisiac, anti-depressant.

● Do not use in pregnancy   ✳ Do not use where skin is exposed to strong sunlight

■ Do not use on sensitive skins   ▲ Do not use with high blood pressure

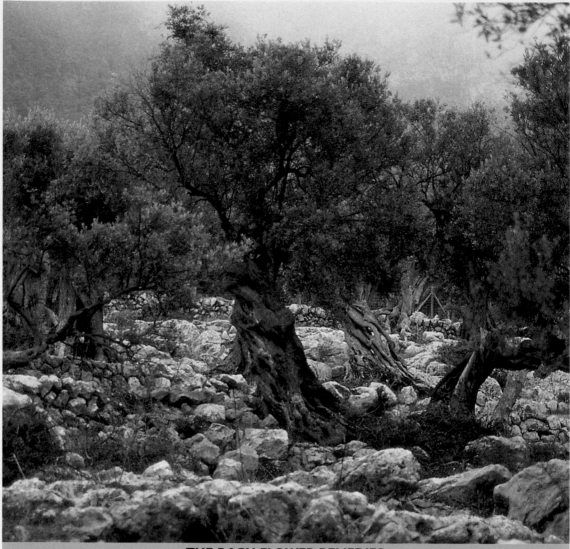

THE BACH FLOWER REMEDIES

Edward Bach was an English physician who practised as a homoeopath in London during the 1920s. He developed a system of remedies based on thirty-seven wild plants, using tinctures prepared from them by infusion or by boiling. His concern was to identify cures for the psychological states of individuals that depleted the immune system.

In some ways his emphasis looked forward to contemporary concern with the effect of the mind on the body. In others it looked back to the medieval Doctrine of Signatures where the appearance or habit of the plant was thought to indicate what it would cure.

AN OLIVE GROVE IN NORTH-WEST MAJORCA.
OLIVE FLOWERS ARE THE BACH REMEDY FOR MENTAL EXHAUSTION.

Botanical name	Common name	Used to treat
Aesculus × carnea	Red Chestnut	Fear for others.
Aesculus hippocastanum	White Chestnut	Worry, with an over-active mind.
Aesculus hippocastanum (bud)	White Chestnut	Slowness in learning.
Agrimonia eupatoria	Agrimony	Worry, when hidden by a cheerful façade.
Bromus ramosus	Wild Oat	Lack of direction.
Calluna vulgaris	Ling	Fear of loneliness in those self-absorbed.
Carpinus betulus	Hornbeam	Fear of lack of strength in daily duties.
Castanea sativa	Sweet Chestnut	Anguish in those exhausted.
Centaurium umbellatum	Centaury	Those who give in too much to the demands of others.
Ceratostigma willmottianum	Plumbago	Indecision.
Cichorium intybus	Chicory	Possessiveness, in those critical of others.
Clematis vitalba	Old Man's Beard	Those who are not rooted in the present and tend to dream.
Fagus sylvatica	Beech	Intolerance.
Gentiana amarella*	Felwort	Self-doubt.
Helianthemum nummularium	Rock Rose	Terror.
Hottonia palustris	Water Violet	Reticence, over self-reliance.
Ilex aquifolium	Holly	For jealousy, envy, desire for revenge.
Impatiens glandulifera	Impatiens	Irritability, impatience.
Juglans regia	Walnut	Those distracted by others from their own life aims.
Larix decidua	Larch	Lack of self-confidence and fear of failure.
Lonicera caprifolium	Honeysuckle	Those who look back too much to happier days.
Malus pumila	Crab Apple	Those who feel unclean.
Mimulus guttatus	Monkey Flower	Phobias.
Olea europaea	Olive	Mental prostration.
Ornithogalum umbellatum	Star of Bethlehem	Shock.
Pinus sylvestris	Scots Pine	Self-reproach.
Populus tremula	Aspen	Fears: source unknown.
Prunus cerasifera	Cherry Plum	Fears of insanity or senility.
Quercus robur	English Oak	Depression, in those who battle courageously.
Rosa canina	Wild Rose	Apathy.
Salix alba var. vitellina	Yellow Willow	Bitterness and resentment.
Scleranthus annuus	Scleranthus	Indecision, without resort to advice.
Sinapsis arvensis	Mustard	Severe, unexplainable depression.
Ulex europaeus	Gorse	Despair.
Ulmus procera	English Elm	Those who feel overburdened by responsibility.
Verbena officinalis	Vervain	Strain in those who are energetic but have fixed ideas.
Vitis vinifera	Grape Vine	Dominance, over-forcefulness.

*There is doubt over which species Bach identified.

For more information contact the Dr Edward Bach Centre,

Mount Vernon, Sotwell, Wallingford, Oxon OX10 0PZ, England.

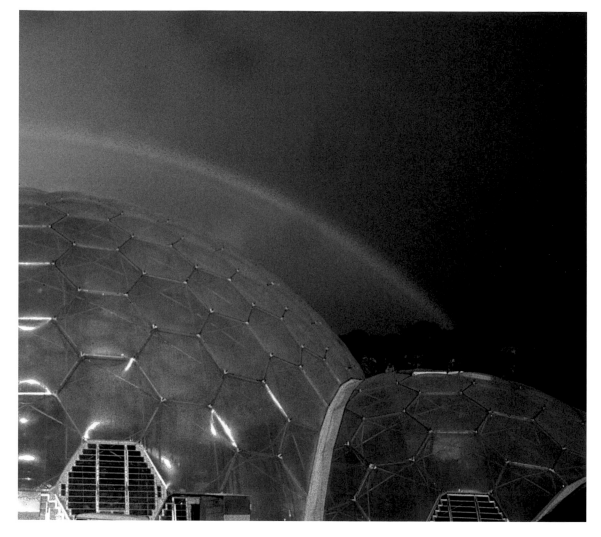

of the water, carbon and nitrogen cycles and, ultimately, of the world's climate. Plants create and drive the atmosphere and are therefore part of the 'self-healing' of planet Earth itself.

The Eden Project has made great efforts to expand people's awareness of their interaction with the plant world from the cultivation of their own gardens to a global view. The importance of taking a broader view is apparent to visitors from the moment they enter; there is an emphasis on the (often inequitable) global distribution of resources as well as on the movement of crops in trading patterns around the world; and what are now termed 'ecosystem services' provided by plants, such as the hydrology cycle, the protection of water catchments and the protection of soils from erosion, are featured and explained as visitors move around the site.

THE EDEN PROJECT INSTILS HOPE FOR THE HEALING OF DAMAGED LANDSCAPES
BY CREATING A GLOBAL GARDEN IN A MINE.

PLANTS AS HEALERS OF LANDSCAPES AND COMMUNITIES

The Eden Project is itself an example of a healed landscape. Before it was clothed in its green mantle of planting, it was a flooded china clay pit, a quarry devoid of soil and vegetation. The response of the public to this 'greening' process, which involved 85,000 tonnes of soil mixes being artificially created, has been enormously positive. No one wants to see mined landscapes exploited and then abandoned. All over the world, good practice in mining is now to restore such landscapes – and to cost that restoration as part of the extraction costs, the 'true' costs.

Eden is also working, with the Cornwall Heathland Project, on the largest landscape recreation plan of its kind in Europe. This involves reshaping large areas of china clay waste tips and recreating heathland for wildlife and local community use. This repair of historic landscapes (in the eighteenth century there were 80,000 hectares of heathland in Cornwall; now there are only 7,000) is having important psychological effects on the local communities. The reinvestment shows that the land has not just been raped until the resource is exhausted and the workers laid off.

Of course, 'restoration ecology', as the new discipline is called, is not limited to restoration of mines and has international potential. Any landscape despoiled by human impact qualifies for treatment. In the late 1990s it was estimated that 43 per cent of the earth's land surface was impaired in its ability to supply benefits to humankind because of recent impacts of land use. Good science now underlies these practices – the use of local sources of seed adapted to the locality, an understanding of 'keystone' species crucial to the functioning of the ecosystem, an understanding of soil structure and soil organisms – all these and more add to the success of schemes.

We know that, within cities, there is an urgent need to repair environments, create gardens from derelict land and encourage pride in the environment. I was once very moved by hearing a black child from one of the bleak, treeless townships outside Cape Town, who had arrived in that city via the Kirstenbosch Botanic Gardens' 'outreach' bus, say, 'Wow, you sure have environment!' In New York, the Bronx 'Green Up' campaign has restored derelict city lots to productive gardens with a positive effect on the local community. In Falmouth in southern Cornwall, not far from Eden, the regeneration of gardens has been a keystone in the programme of improving some rundown housing estates and reducing crime. An address for further information about these issues (Transforming Violence) is given on page 185.

Some plants can help clean up contaminated land by extracting and accumulating toxic metals within their tissues. This process – known as phytoremediation – can turn ill into good both for sites and potentially in the recovery of metals (such as nickel or zinc) for other uses. The plants are both healing the site and acting as a 'miner' of the metals which can then be removed in the laboratory by 'phytoextraction'. Paradoxically, some of the world's rarest plants need these toxic sites to survive – such is the power of plant evolution.

MANAGING THE WORLD'S MEDICINAL PLANT MATERIAL

It is vital to conserve and manage the world's plant resources. While a large majority of the global population still relies on herbalism for its basic health care, many of the plants come from unsustainable sources. It is estimated that 85 per cent of pharmaceutical drugs are in some way linked to a plant source, and 25 per cent of prescriptions in the USA contain a principal ingredient derived from a plant. Plant-related pharmaceutical drugs may rise rather than go down in the foreseeable future, yet plant species are becoming extinct before they can be screened.

The medicinal plant trade

It has been estimated that around 20,000 medicinal herbs are used worldwide, the vast majority harvested from the wild. There are usually herb stalls to be seen in local markets and sometimes vast repositories of plant material are brought from the wild into urban centres, such as Durban, in Kwa Zulu Natal. In Europe the trade is centred in Hamburg with large wholesale warehouses serving well-known high-street retailers. A study in 1997 for the German CITES (Convention on International Trade in Endangered Species of Fauna and Flora) authority showed that 1,560 different herbs were being imported; of these 70–90 per cent were from the wild and only 50–100 products were being propagated and cultivated on a large scale.

Protecting medicinal herbs from over-exploitation is important because they are a necessary resource for 85 per cent of the world's population, as well as a preferred resource for many who can afford pharmaceuticals. It is also important to deter substitution of similar species that could be ineffective at best – or poisonous at worst. Among ways in which stocks of herbs could be better managed, one is through consumer power (the effect of which was proved by Britain's rejection of GM foods); current systems of certification for sustainable harvesting of herbs from the wild include that of the British-based Soil Association, and more source labelling on high-street herbs is likely to develop over the next decade. Another way is through the regulation of the plant trade; under the EU's Traditional Herbal Medicinal Products Directive, importers will have to demonstrate 'full traceability' of products back to the field or hillside, which should concentrate the traders' minds on sustainable production and the value of certification schemes, which cover sustainable 'wild harvesting'.

It is not just known medicinal herbs that need conserving. Since the 1980s there has been a growing awareness of threat to the natural environment by the actions of human beings. Nature is no longer seen as a vast system that remains largely unaffected by what we do. Increasing evidence has shown the destruction of the protective ozone layer by chlorofluorocarbons, along with worrying indications of climate change, and the pollution and over-abstraction of ground water.

WOMEN TRADING IN MEDICINAL PLANTS IN MENGHAN, YUNNAN PROVINCE, CHINA. THE CHINESE CULTIVATE MANY PLANTS BUT WORLDWIDE, MOST HERBS ARE WILD-COLLECTED.

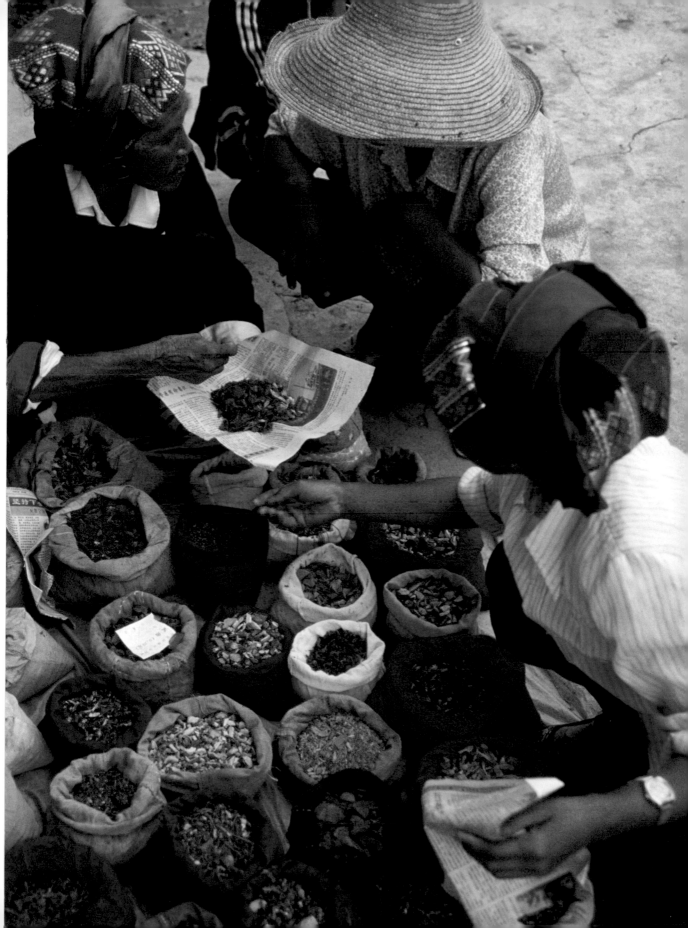

NEW TECHNOLOGIES AND PLANT-BASED DRUGS

In 1992 the so-called 'Earth Summit' in Rio de Janeiro caused a sea change in our attitudes to technologies based on natural materials, including plant-based drugs. Under the terms of the treaty that ensued, the Convention on Biological Diversity, plant material was no longer deemed to be the 'common heritage of human kind'. Instead, it was deemed to be owned by the country in which it originated, forming part of that country's biological wealth, and which the country had a right to exploit, or agree or deny to exploitation by others.

If exploitation rights were granted, the donor country would receive an equitable share of the resultant benefits. Essentially this was a conservation treaty between pharmaceutical companies (based mainly in the Northern hemisphere) and the (usually poor) countries of the South, where much of the biological diversity of the world is held. The deal was 'You conserve your biological heritage rather than destroy it, and we will help you develop its value and share it with you.'

The jury is still out on whether this approach will work in the case of plant-based drugs, because a principal non-ratifier of the treaty is the USA. Most natural-product-biased pharmaceutical companies are now based in the USA, and the 1990s saw a rash of products based closely on 'naturals' being patented there. Some of these patents, for example for drugs based on neem (*Azardirachta indica*) and turmeric (*Cucuma longa*), were challenged successfully by the Indian government on the grounds that knowledge about the use of the plants was widespread in Ayurvedic medicine, i.e. their use was 'not novel'.

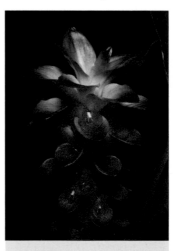

TURMERIC IN FLOWER. THE RHIZOMES HAVE TRADITIONAL MEDICINAL USE AND PATENTS ON THESE HAVE BEEN SUCCESSFULLY CHALLENGED.

Today, reputable companies either work on the flora of their own country, or they attempt to work within the requirements of the Convention on Biological Diversity. This is not always easy, as every country has different rules on access (if any rules have been drawn up) and difficulties arise in places where the government is not recognized by the indigenous peoples from whom the plants are sourced.

A classic example of this dilemma is that of a new class of anti-obesity drug identified by a British company called Phytopharm. Phytopharm learnt of an appetite-suppressant, made from *Hoodia ruschii*, used by the San people of the Kalahari and Botswana during their prolonged hunting expeditions. An extract of *Hoodia* called P57 was licensed to Phytopharm by South Africa's Council

THE PLANT BEING EXAMINED (OPPOSITE) IS *HOODIA RUSCHII*, APPETITE-SUPPRESSANT FOR THE SAN BUSHMAN OF THE KALAHARI AND A POTENTIAL ANTI-OBESITY DRUG.

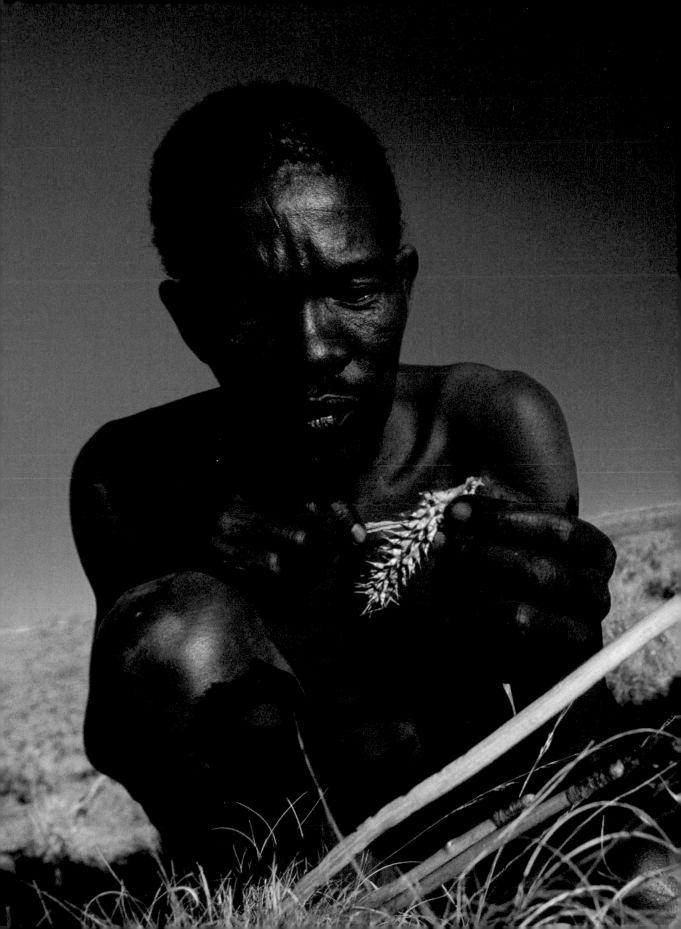

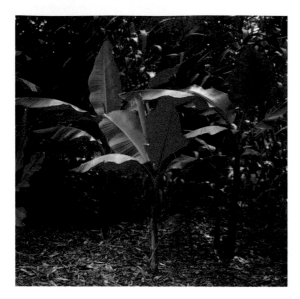

for Scientific and Industrial Research, and production was licensed to Pfizer; the problem was how to return the benefits to the San. With the help of an intermediary, terms were finally agreed and accepted by the community, which also retained the rights to use *Hoodia* in its traditional form. However, Pfizer have now withdrawn from commercialization.

Underlying these controversies are important questions that are likely to be revisited as biotechnology in medicine develops in the new millennium. Who benefits from new therapies from natural materials? Are new therapies mainly developed for 'diseases of the rich' (cancer, coronary heart disease) who can pay for prescriptions rather than 'diseases of the poor' (parasitic diseases) who can't pay? Should natural materials be patentable?

More controversies surround genetic manipulation of crops – the transfer of genes either from one plant species to another, or from other

organisms, such as bacteria, to plants. Developed in the 1980s and 1990s and mainly applied to agriculture, GM technology is now hugely unpopular, particularly in Europe and Japan. In Britain, the Soil Association adheres strongly to the view that the genetic improvement of crops is best done by conventional breeding using genetic marker technology rather than by GM. There is a potential, however, for crops to be designed for all sorts of health benefits: grains with gluten removed, peanuts with allergens removed, bean crops with anti-nutrition factors removed, and so on. There is also the potential to use micro-organisms to achieve health benefits, including using bacteria to produce dairy products without lactose (for lactose-intolerant consumers), soy products without raffinose (which reduces flatulence), low-energy products for the obese (which have non-metabolizable sugars), or to produce substances such as folic acid to reduce the incidence of spina bifida and coronary disease. Only time will tell whether any of these technologies will take off, or whether these products will prove more attractive to consumers than the first generation of GM crops, which were designed to benefit farmers and agrochemical companies.

'Pharming' is another application of genetic engineering. It involves harnessing the ability of plants to produce proteins and using that ability to produce drugs and vaccines within the plant itself. Both herbalists and pharmaceutical chemists know that plants are like chemical factories which produce substances that can be enlisted to fight human disease. The new millennium has brought more interest in plants as 'biorefineries'.

IN THE FUTURE MEDICINAL PRODUCTS MAY BE 'PHARMED' IN PLANTS –
INCLUDING CYSTIC FIBROSIS VACCINES IN BANANAS.

The reason is that the source of most of the synthetic pharmaceuticals produced today, even those where the chemical structure is copied from a plant, is dead plant material (i.e. coal and the petrochemicals derived from it), and supplies are limited. What will happen to medicine when coal and oil reserves run out? Finding the answer is a major motive for looking to living plants to produce drugs and vaccines.

The technology is already with us: diabetics inject insulin from GM bacteria and hepatitis B vaccine uses GM yeast. The latent possibilities are endless. Plants can produce a very great range of proteins accurately, in volume, and potentially cheaply. The last attribute is particularly important. In vaccine production, cost reduction is of the essence if infectious disease (the most common cause of death worldwide) is to be reduced, especially in the developing world. The World Health Organization is looking for a vaccine cost of one dollar a dose including the cost of needle and syringe. Current costs are often twelve times that level and current production from animal or human sources cannot deliver the volume needed for worldwide programmes.

In most cases all plant material will be removed from the product, leaving it identical to that produced by different methods, and either swallowed as a pill or injected as with conventional vaccines.

What are the concerns here? Will the overriding fear of GM prevail and opposition spread to this brave new world of vaccines from plants? Will using plants as bioreactors be seen as more ethically acceptable than using animals?

There is some evidence that the public are more receptive to high-tech techniques in medicine than in food production. In terms of safety, the regulatory regimes for testing pharmaceuticals are far more rigorous than for foods; there is perhaps reason to trust plants more than animals, because plants are not affected by viruses and bacteria (and the prion that causes the human form of BSE), which affect animals and could spread infection. Drug and vaccine production in plants is likely to take place mainly in contained environments in glasshouses. Even when larger quantities of pharmed crops are needed, for example, for AIDS, TB and malaria, they would be grown on a far smaller scale than food crops, with fewer environmental risks though still of concern to some ('Will I be eating someone's prescription drugs from the maize in my cornflakes?').

Only time will tell what the future will bring; at present, pharmaceutical companies have yet to embrace these new possibilities. When Charles Jenner began smallpox vaccination using serum from cows there was widespread fear that people would start developing udders. Vaccination is now widely accepted and has eliminated some diseases. What is feared today may be commonplace tomorrow.

Future products

What sort of products will there be and what will they be like? Recent investigations have included:

a measles vaccine from tobacco

antibiotics for cancers from tobacco (these are known as 'plantbiotics')

cystic fibrosis vaccines from bananas

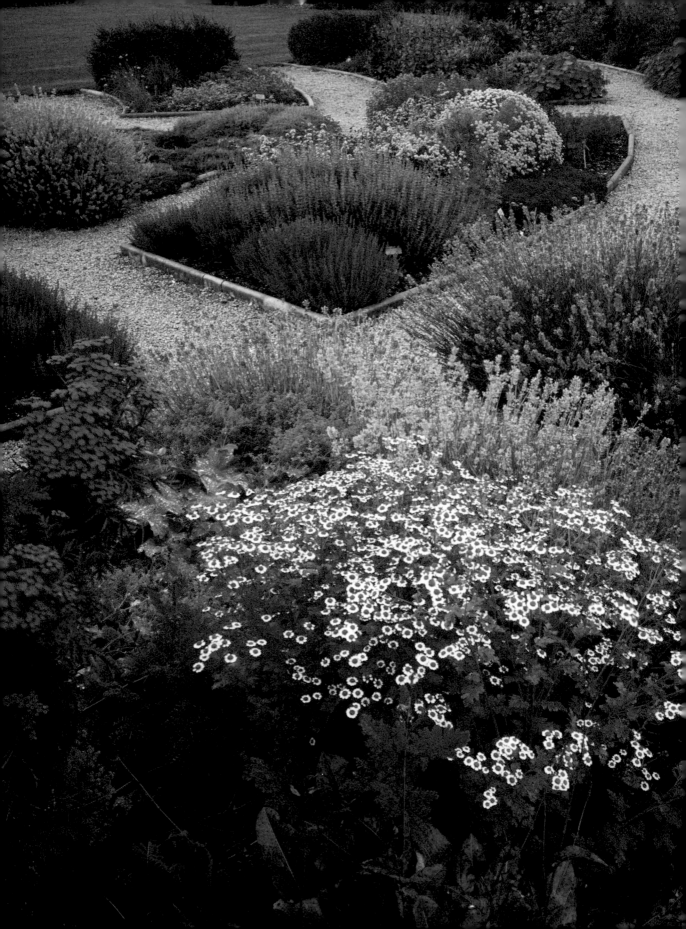

NATURE'S
PHARMACY

THERE ARE SOME PLANTS FROM THE WIDE
CATALOGUE OF NATURE'S PHARMACY THAT ARE USEFUL
AS REMEDIES FOR MINOR AILMENTS; MORE ARE OF
GREAT IMPORTANCE IN TODAY'S PHARMACEUTICAL
and food supplement industries, and many also make very good
garden plants, being easy to grow and attractive to look at. The
merits of eating fresh fruit and vegetables, for the nutritious
vitamins, minerals, fibre and antioxidants they contain, are
now known to be more important than ever. A greater range of
all these plants – whether shrubs, perennials, annuals, fruit
trees or vegetable varieties – is becoming widely available,
making it possible to create a garden that is both ornamental
and a source of good health.

THIS ORNAMENTAL GARDEN CONTAINS LAVENDERS, HIGHLY POPULAR IN AROMATHERAPY
AND (FOREGROUND) FEVERFEW WHICH IS A HERBAL REMEDY FOR MIGRAINE.

MEDICINAL HERBS

There are a number of herbs that are simple to cultivate and can be safely used as remedies for common ailments. (The term 'herb' refers here to any plant material used for medicinal purposes.) Herbal treatments, sometimes called phytomedicines, have been tried and tested over the years and can have beneficial effects, but it is important that only minor problems are self-treated; if an ailment is severe or persists, you should seek help from a qualified medical practitioner because the condition may be a more deep-seated illness. You should also be aware that some herbal medicines interact with pharmaceutical drugs, so you should always tell your doctor if you are taking herbal remedies.

A GLOSSARY OF TREATMENT METHODS

These are the main methods of treatment used in traditional folk medicine, in over-the-counter preparations (sold without a doctor's prescription) and as dispensed by medical herbalists.

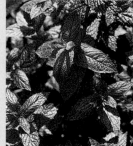

Compress

Lint or cotton wool dipped into a herbal infusion (see below) and applied externally. Compresses can be applied hot or (more commonly) cold to reduce bruising etc. External herbal treatment by compress was common in many traditions of ethnic medicine.
(See also Poultice opposite.)

Decoction

The liquid produced when a herb is boiled and imparts its healing properties to the liquid.

Infusion

The liquid produced when a herb has been covered with boiling water for several minutes. This is the commonest method of producing a herbal tea, but some are made by decoction (see above).

Oil

The mixture produced when a herb has infused its potency into vegetable oil and a small amount of vinegar over a period of weeks in a warm place. These oils can be used in therapeutic massage.

Ointment

A paste for external application produced by adding crushed herbs to melted petroleum jelly and simmering for about twenty minutes.

Poultice

A soft, hot mixture of fresh herbs briefly boiled in muslin and applied externally. Poultices are commonly used in many traditions of ethnic medicine.

Syrup

The result of adding sugar to a herbal infusion and simmering until the consistency is syrupy. Often used for minor ailments in children as a more palatable medicine.

Tincture

A herbal extract preserved in alcohol in which it will keep indefinitely. Tinctures are the commonest method of prescription by medical herbalists.

PEPPERMINT IS ONE OF THE COMMONEST HERBS USED
TO MAKE A HERBAL TEA OR INFUSION.

Agrimonia eupatoria Agrimony

This perennial herb reaches 60 × 30cm (24 × 12in) and bears spikes of small yellow flowers in summer. It is easily raised from seed. Grow it in the border or a wildflower meadow in dry, limey soils. When infused, agrimony will form a useful gargle for throat infections and mild catarrh. *Hardiness zone 8.*

Aloe vera Aloe

A frost-tender succulent, aloe will grow to 60cm (24in) on a sunny window sill and, like most succulents, it needs well-drained, sandy compost and to dry out between waterings. Directly applied, the gel from the leaves is a useful 'first aid' for minor burns or mild sunburn: just break off a leaf and cut it open. The main active ingredient is allantoin. *Hardiness zone 8.*

Althaea officinalis Marshmallow

This perennial with soft, lobed leaves typical of the mallow family, and pale pink flowers, grows rapidly to 90cm–1.2m (3–4ft). It can be grown from spring-sown seed or from cuttings. It will succeed in any soil, but will grow more luxuriantly in rich, moist conditions. In herbal medicine the roots and leaves are used in compresses to reduce inflammation, and as an infusion for coughs and chest infections. *Hardiness zone 3.*

Calendula officinalis Marigold

Pot marigolds are annuals easily raised from seed. They quickly reach 30cm (12in) and produce yellow and orange flowers all summer. They need sun but tolerate any well-drained soil. They have

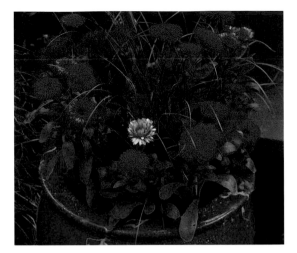

a multitude of uses in healing. For dry skin, infuse the flowers in boiling water for twenty minutes, and when cool, strain and apply the infusion to the skin. This infusion will also heal an inflamed digestive tract when taken internally. When formed into an ointment, calendula is one of the most widely used dry skin creams. *Hardiness zone 6.*

Chamaemelum nobile Roman chamomile *and Matricaria recutita* German chamomile

Roman chamomile is a perennial, prostrate plant, often used to create chamomile lawns or seats (especially using the cultivar 'Treneague'); German chamomile is an annual growing to 30cm (12in). Both these species are aromatic foliage plants with flowers that are used medicinally. The flowers are infused as a tea (the German form is generally less bitter), and used to induce sleep and calm digestive upsets. Both species prefer light soil in full sun, and can be raised from seed ('Treneague' must be obtained from cuttings). *Hardiness zone 4 and 7, respectively.*

MARIGOLD (*CALENDULA OFFICINALIS*) IS MAINLY USED IN HEALING THE SKIN
AND IS AN EXCELLENT MOISTURIZER.

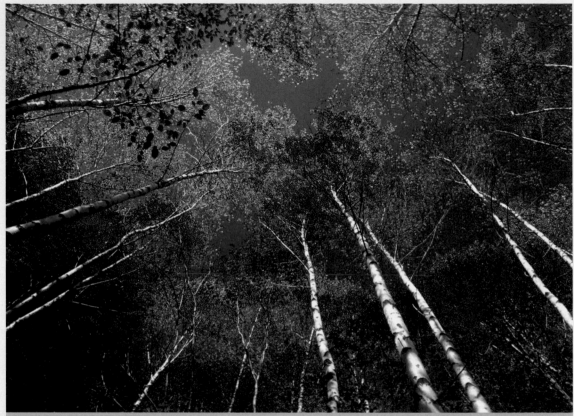

THE PLANT ORIGINS OF SOME MAJOR MODERN DRUGS

There are a number of important drugs that owe their origin directly to a plant. In some cases the active ingredient from the plant is used directly (artemisinin, digoxin, vincristine, atropine and morphine). In others, the plant ingredient provides the basis upon which a part-synthetic drug is developed (etoposide). In some cases discovery of the active ingredient has led to the development of a synthetic drug (contraceptive steroids are now synthesized rather than extracted from yams). Chemists have also copied how a plant's secondary compounds work and have developed a more reliable synthetic drug (dicoumarol).

Of the latest developments in pharmaceutical drug research, watch out for:

- neck and throat cancer drugs from *Combretum caffrum*, a South African tree (combretastatin)

- new drugs for difficult leukaemias from *Cephalotaxus harringtonia*, a Chinese conifer (homoharringtonine), and from *Indigofera tinctoria*

- melanoma treatments from *Betula alba* (betulinic acid)

- potential new antimalarial drugs from the Cameroon vine (*Ancistrocladus korupensis*) (michellamine B)

BETULINIC ACID FROM BIRCH IS A POTENTIAL NEW PHARMACEUTICAL TREATMENT FOR MELANOMA.

Drug	Medical use	Plant source
Amiodarone	For heartbeat irregularity.	*Ammi visnaga*
Artemisinin	For malaria.	*Artemisia annua*
Aspirin	As a painkiller.	*Filipendula ulmaria*, Meadowsweet
Atropine	To stimulate the heart during heart attack.	*Atropa belladonna*, Deadly Nightshade
Camptothecin	For colo-rectal cancer.	*Camptotheca acuminata*
Carbenoxalone	For peptic ulcer.	*Glycyrrhiza glabra*, Liquorice
Cocaine	As a painkiller.	*Erythroxylum coca*, Coca
Codeine	As a painkiller.	*Papaver somniferum*, Opium Poppy
Colchicine	For gout.	*Colchicum autumnale*, Meadow Saffron
Dicoumarol	As an anticoagulant to prevent thrombosis.	*Melilotus officinalis*, Melilot
Digoxin	To strengthen and normalize heartbeat.	*Digitalis lanata*, Woolly Foxglove
Ephedrine	Nasal decongestant.	*Ephedra* species
Etoposide	For various cancers.	*Podophyllum peltatum*, American Mandrake
Galanthamine	For Alzheimer's disease.	*Narcissus* bulbs
Hyoscine and Hyoscyamine	As a relaxant before major anaesthesia; for motion sickness.	*Mandragora officinarum*, Mandrake, but commercially from *Duboisia myoporoides*
Lignocaine	As a local anaesthetic.	*Hordeum vulgare*, Barley
Methoxsalen	For skin cancer, psoriasis and vitiligo.	*Ammi majus*
Morphine	As an excellent painkiller.	*Papaver somniferum*, Opium Poppy
Nifedipine	For angina and hypertension.	*Ammi visnaga*
Physostigmine	For paralysis in myasthenia gravis and for glaucoma.	*Physostigma venenosum*, Ordeal Bean
Pilocarpine	For glaucoma.	*Pilocarpus microphyllus*, jaborandi
Quinidine	For irregular heartbeat.	*Cinchona* spp., Quinine
Quinine	For malaria and muscle cramps.	*Cinchona* spp., Quinine
Salicin	As a painkiller and anti-rheumatic.	*Salix* spp., Willow
Steroids (including contraceptives)	To reduce inflammation and to prevent conception.	*Agave sisalana*, Sisal, and *Dioscorea* spp., Yam
Taxol	For uterine and breast cancer.	*Taxus baccata*
Theophylline	To reduce excess blood formation after kidney transplantation; as a diuretic.	*Camellia sinensis*, Tea
Tubocurarine	As a muscle relaxant.	*Chondrodendron tomentosum*, Curare
Vincristine and Vinblastine	For leukaemia and Hodgkin's disease.	*Catharanthus roseus*, Rosy Periwinkle

MEDICINAL PLANTS FOR ORNAMENT

There is quite a range of plants used either in traditional herbalism or as drug plants in orthodox medicine that are very ornamental in their own right. All the following species could be used to create a specialist area in your own garden, or in the green-house. You might try using the woody species, such as hawthorn, witch hazel, elder and rose, as the main structural planting and then infill with the perennials. Leave spaces for some of the fast-growing annuals, such as the opium poppy, melilot and artemisia, which can be sown outdoors in spring. Especially if you are planning to grow these plants in a border, it is worth noting their mature heights so that you can plant the highest at the back and grade them so that the shortest is in the front. For extra height, particularly when the woody species are young and small, you can train the hop onto a tripod of stakes or an ornamental iron column.

Achillea millefolium Yarrow

This perennial, which is native to Britain, has feathery foliage and white, flattened heads of flowers throughout summer. It grows to 60cm (2ft) and spreads vigorously (some would say it is weedlike), self-seeding very freely. There is a pink variety called 'Cerise Queen'. John Parkinson's *Paradisus* of 1629 recommended it for staunching bleeding, and it was used for this purpose in emergency during the First World War. Yarrow can be made into an ointment for chilblains. *Hardiness zone 2.*

Artemisia annua

This annual member of the daisy family can be raised from seed sown direct into the ground in spring. It grows to about 90cm (3ft) and produces attractive feathery leaves and short spikes of insignificant flowers in late summer. It has been used for centuries in China to treat malaria, and artemisinin extracted from it is now used to treat cerebral malaria, which is resistant to treatment by synthetic drugs. *Hardiness zone 8.*

Capsicum annuum Chilli pepper

Chillies are annuals which grow to about 60cm (24in) and are highly ornamental in pots. They are a source of the analgesic capsaicin. *Hardiness zone 9.*

Centaurium erythraea Centaury

This biennial is a native of English chalk down-lands and needs poor, limey soil to do well. From a rosette of leaves at the base, the flower stems grow to 30cm (12in) (often less) and produce panicles of pink flowers. This bitter herb has been used in herbal medicine to relieve gout, and to stimulate the liver and digestion. *Hardiness zone 8.*

Colchicum autumnale Meadow saffron

This bulbous plant flowers in the late summer and early autumn, producing lilac flowers similar

THE MALE FERN, *DRYOPTERIS FILIX-MAS* (RIGHT, CENTRE), WAS ONCE USED AS A HERBAL TREATMENT FOR WORMS.

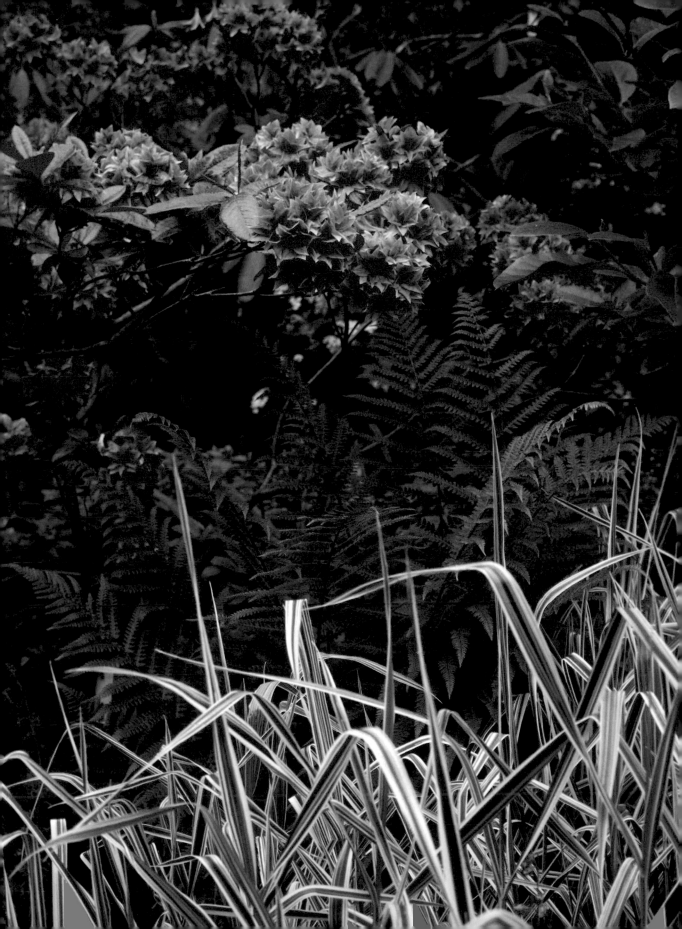

and ephemeral flowers in a range of pinks, either single or double-flowered. The seedpods are harvested to turn into morphine, codeine or papaverine. The plant seeds freely and you may need to remove most of the pods before they ripen to restrict self-seeding. Dried, the pods make excellent indoor decorations. *Hardiness zone 7.*

Podophyllum hexandrum Indian mandrake and *Podophyllum peltatum* American mandrake

These herbaceous perennials need a rich moist soil and some shade. They have ephemeral pinkish flowers followed by large scarlet fruits and are useful for their drooping, deeply cleft, brownish leaves. Neither species grows to more than 30cm (12in). Semi-synthetic drugs based on extracts from the roots are used to treat lung, kidney and testicular cancers. *Hardiness zone 6 and 4, respectively.*

Primula veris Cowslip

The leaves of this spring-flowering perennial British native expand rapidly in early spring in small rosettes from which the heads of yellow scented flowers emerge to reach 15–20cm (6–8in). In herbal medicine this plant was used to treat migraine, especially when taken as cowslip wine, and Culpeper recommended it for acne and other skin eruptions. Modern herbalists still use the flowers to relieve tension headaches. Obtain plants from seed or as plugs – never take them from the wild. *Hardiness zone 5.*

Rheum palmatum Chinese or Ornamental rhubarb

This perennial plant is a relative of the common or garden rhubarb (*R. rhaponticum*), and originates from China, where its roots have been used to treat both constipation and dysentery. It is useful for its dramatic foliage and will easily grow to 1.5m (5ft) in good, moist soil, producing panicles of red flowers in midsummer. *Hardiness zone 6.*

Rosa Rose

The main species of rose used medicinally are *Rosa × damascena*, the damask rose (*hardiness zone 4*), and *R. × centifolia*, the cabbage rose (*hardiness zone 5*). Both are used in perfumery and aromatherapy for their scent. *R. canina*, the wild English dog rose (*hardiness zone 3*), produces scarlet hips which are used in rose hip syrup, an excellent source of vitamin C. It is rarely planted in gardens (except in wild gardens) however, because of its brief flowering period. *R. gallica* (*hardiness zone 5*) was used to produce astringent rose water, while *R. gallica* 'Officinalis' became known as the apothecaries' rose because it was used widely in French folk medicine to treat sore throats and diarrhoea. *R. gallica* 'Officinalis' has a rather harsh red and white flower said to symbolize the settlement of the medieval Wars of the Roses and is therefore a symbol of peace. All these roses need full sun. *Hardiness zone 5.*

Scutellaria lateriflora Skullcap

This (and other species of skullcap) were long thought to help 'head' diseases but are now used in herbal medicine for nervous exhaustion. This perennial grows to 60–90cm (2–3ft) and needs moist soil. The flowers are blue and helmet-shaped like medieval skullcaps. *Hardiness zone 8.*

ROSA X DAMASCENA 'TRIGINTIPETALA' (OPPOSITE) IS THE KAZANLIK ROSE, VITAL TO THE ROSE OIL INDUSTRY OF TURKEY.

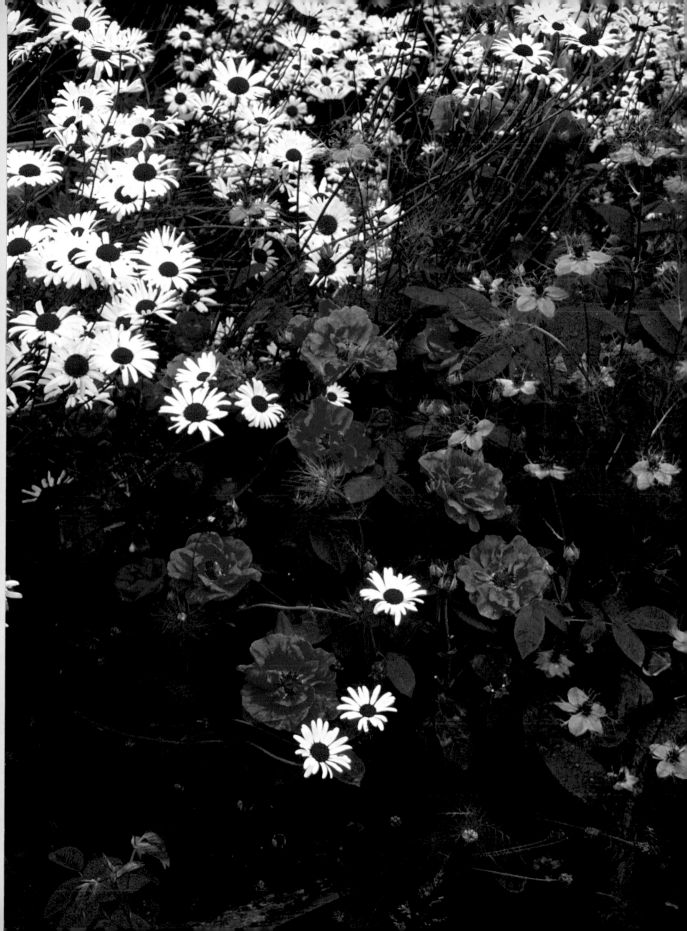

MEDICINAL PLANTS TO GROW INDOORS
OR IN THE CONSERVATORY

Camellia sinensis Tea

Tea plants are sometimes available as conservatory plants. Like most tender camellias, they need to be kept frost-free, in light shade and in moisture-retentive compost. They can reach 1–4m (3–12ft), and produce small white flowers with golden stamens during the winter. The theophylline in tea is used in treating kidney transplant patients and in asthma. *Hardiness zone 8.*

Catharanthus roseus Rosy periwinkle

This perennial is often sold as a pot plant, either in its pink form or in the varieties 'Alba' (a large-flowered pure white) or 'Ocellata' (a white flower with a central pink eye). It can also be grown from seed. It reaches 30cm (12in) and it will flower all the year round, although the flowers are smaller in the winter. It is wise to renew your stock by taking cuttings in spring as the plants can become lanky and do not respond well to being pruned back. The alkaloids this pretty plant contains are extracted from field-grown plants and have cured tens of thousands of children suffering from leukaemia. It is used in a wide variety of cancers. *Hardiness zone 10.*

Gelsemium sempervirens Carolina jasmine

This evergreen climber which reaches 3–6m (10–20ft) comes from the southern USA and needs deep rich soil. It produces its showy yellow flowers in spring. The root is used medicinally in homoeopathy, and has also been used to treat migraine and neuralgia. *Hardiness zone 9.*

Quassia amara

This is a tropical American tree which is occasionally available as a conservatory plant, as it will flower even as a young cutting. The leaves are unusual in having winged stalks with red midribs and the flowers are scarlet. This plant needs to be grown in a warm conservatory and is best in a bed of rich soil. Its bitter bark is used as a tonic and is used, along with the root, against dysentery. *Hardiness zone 10.*

Senna alexandrina Senna

Senna is a shrubby perennial that can be grown from seed (providing you soak the seed in hot water for twenty-four hours before sowing), and will reach 1m (3ft). A member of the pea family, it produces small yellow flowers in the spring and summer even when it is a small plant and may even set the pods favoured in purgative medicine. *Hardiness zone 10.*

Zingiber officinale Ginger

Ginger can be grown as a foliage pot plant from rhizomes, providing these are planted when they are plump and fresh. They need a rich soil and a warm window sill, where they will produce thin leafy shoots that give a fragrance when bruised. Do not hope for flowers as long cycles of vegetative propagation seem to have reduced this plant's ability to produce them. Ginger has been shown to be very effective against travel sickness and morning sickness in pregnancy. *Hardiness zone 10.*

THE ROSY PERIWINKLE (*CATHARANTHUS ROSEUS*) IS FIELD-CROPPED FOR ALKALOIDS TO
COUNTER LEUKAEMIA, HODGKIN'S DISEASE AND MANY CANCERS.

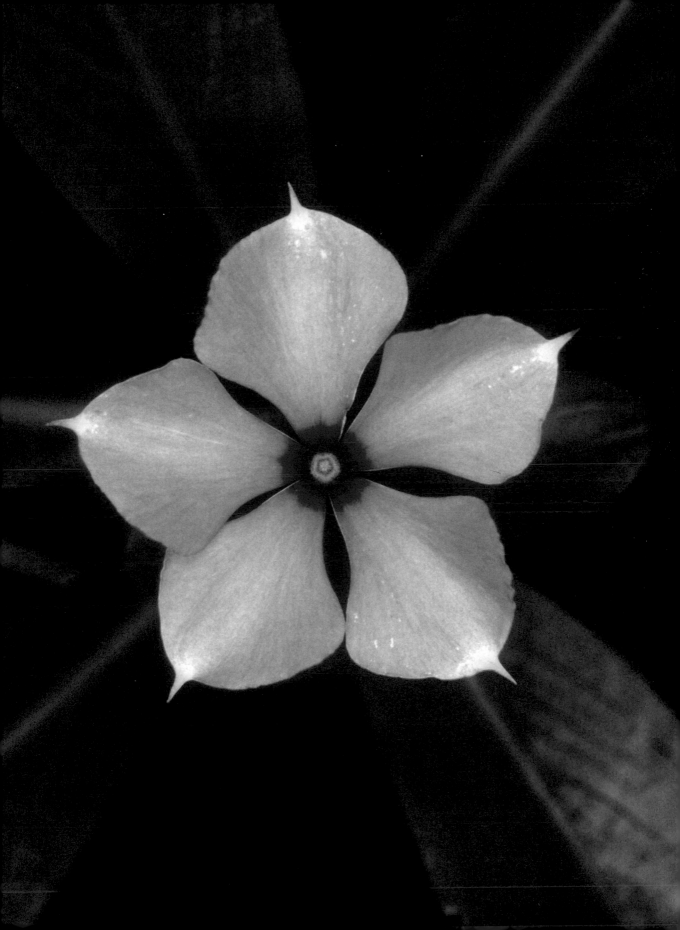

HEALTHY EATING

'**Y**ou are what you eat' is now an accepted idea in the West. But in fact it is a relatively new concept, and indeed the entire science of nutrition and the metabolism of food in the body only developed in the West in the early twentieth century. This is much later than in other areas of the world; in India, for example, diet has always been integral to the ancient Ayurvedic code of healing. It is estimated that 60 per cent of deaths in 2004 were from heart disease, cancers and diabetes. All these diseases have a dietary component and with expectations that the percentage of deaths from these may rise to 73 per cent by 2020, it is little wonder that the debates about food and its effects on health have moved centre stage.

The 1980s and 1990s brought a concern about the effects of synthetic food colourants and food additives, and especially possible links between these and hyperactivity in children. The new millennium has brought concern about soaring levels of obesity, particularly in children, as calorie levels increase and activity levels decrease. Globally, 300 million adults, including 115 million in developing countries, are said to be obese. The highest rates are in the USA, where one-third of adults are clinically obese. The diets of many Americans and Northern Europeans are currently thought to be too high in sugar, salt, saturated fats and protein, and too low in unsaturated fats, some carbohydrates and fibre, the worst items meriting the epithet 'junk food'. Many ready-made or quickly prepared convenience foods are also high in salt, which can aggra-

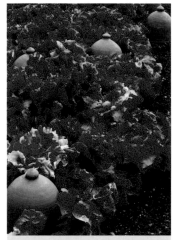

BLANCHING ENDIVES WITH POTS THAT EXCLUDE LIGHT REDUCES THE PLANTS' BITTERNESS.

vate hypertension (high blood pressure). In 2004 the World Health Organization produced a draft strategy to combat obesity and related dietary disease. It recommended lower intakes of sugar, salt and saturated fats, controls on the marketing of junk foods to children, and the use of tax and price policies to influence food consumption.

Dietary concern with fat levels is being rapidly augmented by an awareness of the beneficial effects of fresh fruit and vegetables. In 2003 the British government launched its '5 a day' campaign to encourage people to eat five portions of fresh fruit and vegetables each day, because epidemiological studies suggest that this level of consumption reduces the instances of cancers and coronary disease (the prime killers in the West). The beneficial effect is presumed to come from the antioxidants that

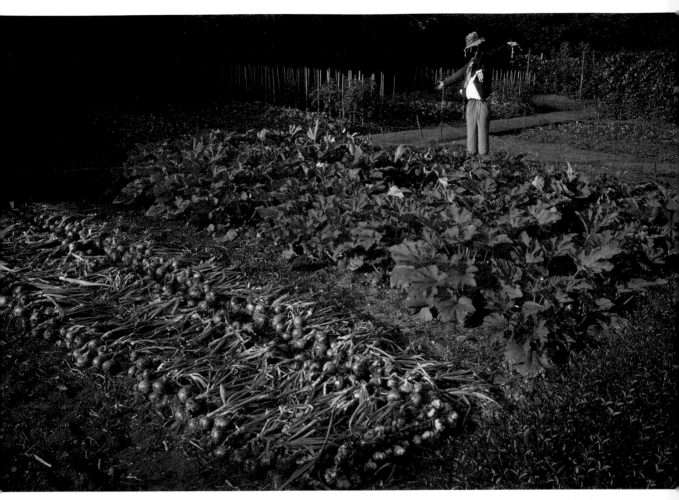

occur naturally in fruit and vegetables. Molecules called free radicals are produced in all of us as a result of respiration. They damage our cells and age us unless 'mopped up' and neutralized by antioxidants.

Despite the statistics of diet-related disease, and the efforts to publicize guidelines to healthier eating, the demand for convenience food continues to grow and manufacturers are ever more adept at marketing foods tailored to the latest food fad. One of the recent commercial responses to the quest for better health from a quick fix rather than a good, balanced diet has been the emergence of 'nutraceuticals'. These are products that combine the roles of nutrition in food and the healing effect of a pharmaceutical drug. They are sometimes called functional foods and are essentially processed, 'supplemented' foods claiming defined health benefits. They are controversial because they challenge regulatory regimes – are they foods or are they medicines? – and because of the high prices that they

GROWING VEGETABLES ON AN ALLOTMENT GARDEN IS A GOOD WAY TO KEEP FIT.
THE ONIONS AND COURGETTE PLANTS SHOWN HERE WOULD FEED A FAMILY OF SIX.

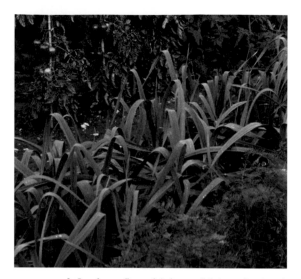

command for benefits which could be obtained more cheaply by a good diet.

In general, foods that have ingredients added for a medical or physiological effect carry a health claim. The most widely marketed functional foods are those relating to obesity, the health of the digestive system, osteoporosis and cancers (the World Health Organization believes that over 35 per cent of cancers are diet-related). In the UK, USA and parts of Europe, particularly Finland, there are large markets in spreading fats that have been modified to reduce blood cholesterol levels. Plant stanol esters found naturally in cereals like rye, wheat and maize are among ingredients used to reduce LDL cholesterol (which causes arterial disease). The fortification of foods with minerals – especially calcium for bone health – has long been a feature of snack grain bars and particularly breakfast cereals. Vitamins are sometimes added to milk and there is an expanding range of drinks fortified with cancer-preventing antioxidants such as vitamins

A, C and E, or with herbal extracts of various sorts including those that are sources of caffeine.

Health claims for these products must stop short of medicinal claims, i.e. claims to 'cure' or 'prevent' disease; but this is inevitably a grey area which codes of practice will need to define. In the UK there is a Code of Practice on Health Claims on Foods, but the standards vary in the UK, Europe and the USA.

One of the longest-running controversies in the debate on food and health has been the discovery of the relation between over-saturated fat and arterial disease. Studies of natural patterns of health have revealed high rates of heart disease among populations with high intakes of animal fats, which in turn have fuelled a move towards vegetarianism.

Fibre in food is considered essential in maintaining good digestive health so there is a need to move towards eating more raw fruit and raw, lightly steamed or stir-fried vegetables and high-fibre cereals – a diet that is much closer to Chinese and Asian traditions. Indeed, studies of Chinese and Japanese immigrants to the USA have shown that they suffer Western rates of heart disease and cancer within one or two generations, through changed diet.

Vegetarianism has also been boosted in more recent years by revulsion against modern methods of factory farming of animals for meat and fish, both on moral and health grounds. There is growing suspicion about the use of growth-stimulating hormones and the residues from regular dosing with antibiotics made necessary by intensive stocking.

GOOD GARDENERS KEEP A SUCCESSION GOING – CROPPING TOMATOES
WHILE LOOKING AHEAD TO THE LEEK CROP ...

ORGANIC GARDENING

Fear of the long-term effects of the residues of pesticides and herbicides in fruit and vegetables has concerned enough people to stimulate demand for organic produce. (In Britain, most organic food is imported, and so adds to environmentally unfriendly food miles.) Growing your own vegetables and fruit is a satisfying way of producing food that is guaranteed free of harmful residues at an acceptable cost. It involves managing your garden organically, which in turn means not only keeping your fruit and vegetables free from pesticides and herbicides, but also having proper respect for the soil. Soil is not a mere carrier of chemicals, rather it is a complex structure that needs careful husbandry.

Good soil structure is maintained by adding plenty of organic matter such as garden compost or well-rotted farmyard manure. This provides nourishment for the plants, helps to aerate the soil, facilitates both drainage and moisture retention and assists root growth. (How to make compost is described on page 68.) Never walk on your soil when it is wet or else you will cause damage by compacting it. Adding lime or gypsum helps the structure of extremely heavy clay soil.

The pros and cons of digging often cause heated debate among organic gardeners. The 'no dig' school claims that digging is a totally unnatural activity and should be replaced by mulching the soil. On the other hand, anyone who has seen the rampant growth of weeds on landslides and landslips will see that plants do respond to the aeration that soil movement provides. The answer is to know your own soil. If it is light it will probably need minimum digging and a good deal of mulching. Clay-based heavy soils are best dug or rotavated in the early autumn before they get sodden and left rough so that frost action will provide a good surface tilth for spring sowing.

Good composting should be at the heart of any organic gardening system, and it is a simple way of recycling the waste that a garden produces. As well as improving the structure of the soil, garden compost, if applied as a mulch to moist soil, will also suppress weeds and help to retain moisture.

It is important not to confuse the two terms 'garden compost' and 'potting compost'. Potting compost is used for potting plants and can be bought from any garden centre. It consists of ingredients that are sterile so as not to introduce bacterial and fungal diseases or weeds to seedlings and young plants. Potting composts are usually made up of a mixture of sterilized loam, grit or perlite and a dressing of fertilizers and trace elements. In Britain peat-based composts generally are being replaced by 'green waste' (composted organic materials generated by local authorities in bulk) or coconut fibre (coir) based composts to conserve the dwindling peat lands of Britain and Ireland, many of which have been designated Sites of Special Scientific Interest.

GROWING VEGETABLES

The great advantages of growing your own vegetables include not only the speed with which you can get them from garden to table (thus preserving the vitamins and antioxidants rapidly lost in transit to shops) but also the unusual types you can choose to grow – and the fact that you can pick them young, before they have got stringy and tough or too large. Such produce may not be easily available in all shops.

You can also choose to grow organically and know that your produce contains no residues. No one knows if these residues are harmful in accumulation, in combination with one another, and over time, so avoiding them is probably wise. Above all, do not attempt to grow vegetables in the heart of urban areas or near busy roads. The fallout of toxic heavy metals from traffic fumes can be significant, especially on to leafy vegetables. Before you set out to grow your own vegetables, you should be sure that your effort will give you enjoyment, because if you cost the time of your labour, the vegetables you produce will not work out cheaper than you can buy them in the shops; however, producing them will certainly help your fitness.

What you can grow will obviously depend upon the space and site that you have. If you have a small garden, decide which are your favourite vegetables and what you have room for. The commercial production of peas is so good now that you may decide that your space is better used to grow mangetout peas, which anyway are rather expensive in the shops and often represent many 'food miles' in terms of air freight. Root crops such as parsnips, carrots and potatoes take up a lot of ground, so you may decide these are not for you; the exception may be young turnips, because they are difficult to buy as they are usually grown to maturity to feed cattle. They are best if you can grow them fast with a lot of water. Onions grown from sets, and leeks, however, are very productive from a small piece of ground. If you like marrows and squashes, grow the bush varieties rather than the trailers as they are more compact. Make full use of cloches to grow winter-hardy lettuce vari-

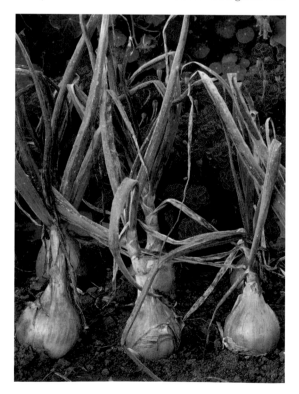

ONIONS CAN BE CLOSELY SPACED, GIVE A HIGH YIELD FROM
A SMALL SPACE, AND CAN BE STORED.

eties and cauliflowers to mature in the spring – these are normally sprayed repeatedly with fungicides by commercial growers. You may be able to grow all your salad requirements in a small space, especially if you sow little and often to avoid a glut.

If you have a small garden you can maximize space by using raised beds which can be accessed by reaching from each side – and therefore cut out the need for spaces between rows. (Row-spacing came about because of the need to accommodate the feet of the gardener.) Raised beds with varieties grown in patches have been shown to be far more productive in yields.

If you have an allotment or large vegetable plot you may be able to produce all you want to eat immediately and enough to store over winter or to freeze. If you want to grow potatoes, you can choose from a range of varieties available as sets to plant in mid spring. Excellent salad varieties include 'Belle de Fontenay' and 'Pink Fir Apple'. The latter is also a particularly good keeper; it can be lifted or harvested in late autumn and stored until the following spring. Commercial varieties of maincrop potatoes are sprayed with maleic hydrazide after harvesting to inhibit them sprouting in store. Tests by the National Vegetable Research Station in Britain (now Horticulture Research International) have shown that pesticides, like vitamins and minerals, are concentrated just under the skin of most vegetables. So by growing your own potatoes you can eat the skins (and get the benefit of the fibre) with peace of mind. The same applies to carrots, which are best peeled to rid them of residues of pesticides sprayed for carrot root fly, unless you have grown your own.

Certain vegetables are grown commercially with very little pesticide simply because breeders have developed good disease-resistant varieties. From the point of view of avoiding residues, therefore, you may not wish to bother growing parsnips, or beetroots for winter storing. Lettuce sold in midsummer has often been grown very fast without artificial fertilizers or pesticides and so is virtually organic. A healthy aphid on such a lettuce is probably a good sign.

Do not exhaust the soil in your vegetable garden by continuous cropping. Rotate your crops according to the pattern shown in the box. If you practise good rotation and soil management you should produce excellent crops organically.

ROTATING YOUR CROPS

Divide the plot into four. Plant potatoes in one section, peas and beans in the second, root vegetables in the third, and cucurbits and brassicas in the fourth. Rotate the cycle each year.

Dig in manure before you plant cucurbits and brassicas. This will be used up by the following year and will not overfeed the root vegetables, which causes them to fork. The peas and beans make their own feed in their roots by taking nitrogen from the air, so need no fertilizers. If you leave their roots in after cropping they will help to feed the succeeding potatoes, although you can augment this by using sterilized fish, blood and bone fertilizer, an excellent organic substitute for the all-purpose chemical fertilizers. The manure is far enough away from the potatoes in the rotation to prevent scab disease.

In this way the vegetable garden feeds itself and the soil is well looked after.

RECOMMENDED VARIETIES OF VEGETABLES

LETTUCE
EARLY VARIETIES
(sown under glass and
transplanted)
'Little Gem'
'Tom Thumb'
MAIN SUMMER
(direct sowings)
Cos varieties
'Valmaire'
'Winter Density'
'Pan's White'
Crispheads
'Iceberg'
'Avoncrisp'
'Webb's Wonderful'
Salad Bowl
(for picking leaves)
'Lollo Rosso'
'Red Oakleaf'
'Cocarde'
OUTDOOR
OVERWINTERING
(sow August)
'Imperial Winter'
'Arctic King'

SALAD ONIONS
'White Lisbon'
'Winter Hardy White
   Lisbon'
'White Sweet Spanish'

ONIONS
FOR SPRING SOWINGS
OR SETS
Storing varieties
'Ailsa Craig'
'Bedfordshire Champion'
'Early Yellow Globe'
Red-fleshed
'Red Baron'
'Southport Red Globe'
FOR AUTUMN SOWINGS
(August) to crop following
spring (or sets)
'Senshyu Semi-Globe
   Yellow'
'Sturon'
'Yellow Granex'

SPINACH
FOR SUMMER SOWINGS
'Dominant'
'Long Standing'
'Matador'
FOR AUTUMN SOWINGS
(winter cropping)
'Green Market'
'Sigmaleaf'

TOMATOES
FOR SMALL SPACES
'Minibel'
'Gardener's Delight'
'Tumbler' (for hanging
baskets)

BEETROOT
EARLY SOWINGS
'Boltardy'
'Regala'
MAIN CROP
'Ruby Queen'
'Vermilion'
'Buyer's Goblin'
   (yellow-fleshed)
'Kugel'

RADISH
'Scarlet Globe'
'White Icicle'
'Sparkler'

CUCURBITS
COURGETTES
'Early Gem'
'Ducato'
'Gold Rush'
MARROWS (compact)
'Rondo de Nice'
'Burpee Golden'
'Sweet Dumpling'
'Minipak'
CUCUMBER
(outdoor, ridge varieties)
'Marketmore'

PEAS
MANGETOUT
'Carouby de Maussane'
'Dwarf White Sugar'
'Oregon Sugar Pod'

SNAP VARIETIES
'Sugar Snap'
'Sugar Daddy'

POTATOES
EARLY VARIETIES
'Arran Pilot'
'Arran Comet'
'Charlotte' (salad)
SECOND EARLY
'Estima'
'Kondor' (red-skinned)
'Ratte' (salad)
'Edzell Blue'
   (blue-skinned)
MAIN CROP
'Desirée' (pink-skinned)
'Pink Fir Apple'
   (pink-skinned) (salad)

CARROTS
FOR EATING YOUNG
'Baby Nantes'
'Baby Orange'
'Minicor'
'Paris Market'
'Parano'

TURNIPS
'Snowball'
'Purple Top Milan'

LEEKS
'Farinto'
'King Richard'

UNUSUAL VEGETABLES

Growing something out of the ordinary can give you a real sense of achievement as well as yield ingredients for more adventurous meals. The following are easy to grow, though the sweet peppers and aubergines do best in a cold frame or under a cloche.

Abelmoschus esculentus Okra

This is quite easy to crop from seed in warm gardens and it produces very beautiful, though ephemeral, flowers before setting the large pods sometimes known as 'Ladies' Fingers'. This rather mucilaginous vegetable is popular in curries, and it has a high ratio of fibre to flesh. Indians know okra as bhindi. It is best treated as an annual by sowing into a well-manured loam well after risk of frost. *Hardiness zone 9.*

Apium graveolens var. *rapaceum* Celeriac or Turnip-rooted celery

This is a useful vegetable to grow if you have heavy soil in which celery will not grow well. The swollen root can be grated and eaten raw in salads with a dressing of lemon juice, or cut up and roasted. It is a good source of fibre. Store the roots over winter in sand in a dry place for use as required. *Hardiness zone 8.*

Asparagus officinalis Asparagus

This is an excellent crop to grow to save money because asparagus is always expensive to buy. However, you need soil that is free of perennial weeds, quite a bit of space to lay out a bed, patience (it takes several years to crop from two-year-old roots) and discipline (it should not be picked after midsummer or you will run down the strength of the plants). If you can manage all this, enjoy it with butter as a delicious source of fibre. Asparagus crowns are best planted 40cm (16in) apart on ridged soil to improve drainage. *Hardiness zone 4.*

Brassicas Rare and various

In addition to sprouts and cabbages, there is a range of unusual varieties grown by the Chinese and used in stir fries. The secret of Chinese greens is to grow them quickly in a moist soil with a lot of water and eat them young. Kohlrabi is another useful variety, sometimes known as turnip-rooted cabbage. Grow this in the same way, and enjoy its nutty flavour when lightly boiled to preserve the vitamins. Most of these brassicas are sensitive to high temperatures and will bolt (run to seed) easily. *Hardiness zone 8.*

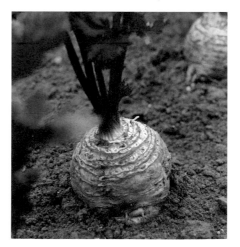

CELERIAC IS A USEFUL SUBSTITUTE FOR CELERY, AND CAN BE STORED, WHICH MAKES IT MORE VERSATILE.

Capsicum annuum Sweet pepper

These require cultivation in a cold greenhouse or under tall cloches, where they are no more diffi-cult to grow than tomatoes, although the seeds need 21°C (70°F) to germinate. They are deli-cious raw or cooked. Use the coloured forms (often marketed as 'traffic light' packs, i.e. in red, yellow and green sequence) to make salads visu-ally appealing. *Hardiness zone 9.*

Crambe maritima Seakale

This is a seaside plant with grey-green leaves and white flowers. If you lift roots in the autumn, pot them up and put them in the dark in an airing cupboard or warm cellar you can force the young shoots. These have a nutty flavour and are a wel-come salad vegetable for the winter when there is a shortage of vitamin-rich fresh produce. Seakale-forcing pots can be used outside to produce blanched shoots. *Hardiness zone 5.*

Cynara scolymus Globe artichoke

This is a thistle-like plant with blue flowers, worthy of a place in the flower border. As a bonus you can cut the unopened flower head and boil it, using the fleshy base of each petal dipped in butter as an appetizer. *Hardiness zone 6.*

Helianthus tuberosus Jerusalem artichoke

This plant produces nutty-flavoured tubers in great profusion, which are an excellent source of fibre and contain a sweetener that can be digested by diabetics. In a good summer the plants will produce flowers like small sunflowers, but beware: each plant is enormously productive.

So do not plant too many or you will have an embarrassment of riches. *Hardiness zone 4.*

Scorzonera hispanica Scorzonera

This is a black-skinned root vegetable with a sweet white flesh digestible by diabetics. If you leave it in the ground for a second season its roots are larger and easier to crop. Sow in open ground in spring. *Hardiness zone 6.*

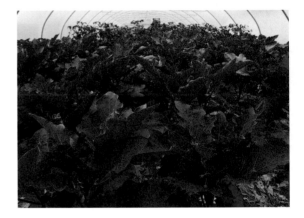

Solanum melongena Aubergine

This is a crop really worth growing under glass in the same way as sweet peppers, and just as easy to grow, providing you introduce a predator against whitefly. Use it chopped and cooked in ratatouille or stuffed and baked with a meat or vegetable fill-ing. It is also an essential ingredient of Greek moussaka. Do not eat aubergines raw. *Hardiness zone 10.*

Tragopogon porrifolius Salsify

This root vegetable is grown in the same way as scorzonera but tastes somewhat like oysters. It is sometimes known as the vegetable oyster. It is very good in a creamed soup. *Hardiness zone 5.*

AUBERGINES GROW WELL IN POLYTUNNELS (ABOVE) AS THEY ENJOY EXTRA HEAT AND HUMIDITY.
KOHLRABI (OPPOSITE) IS BEST EATEN YOUNG AND TENDER.

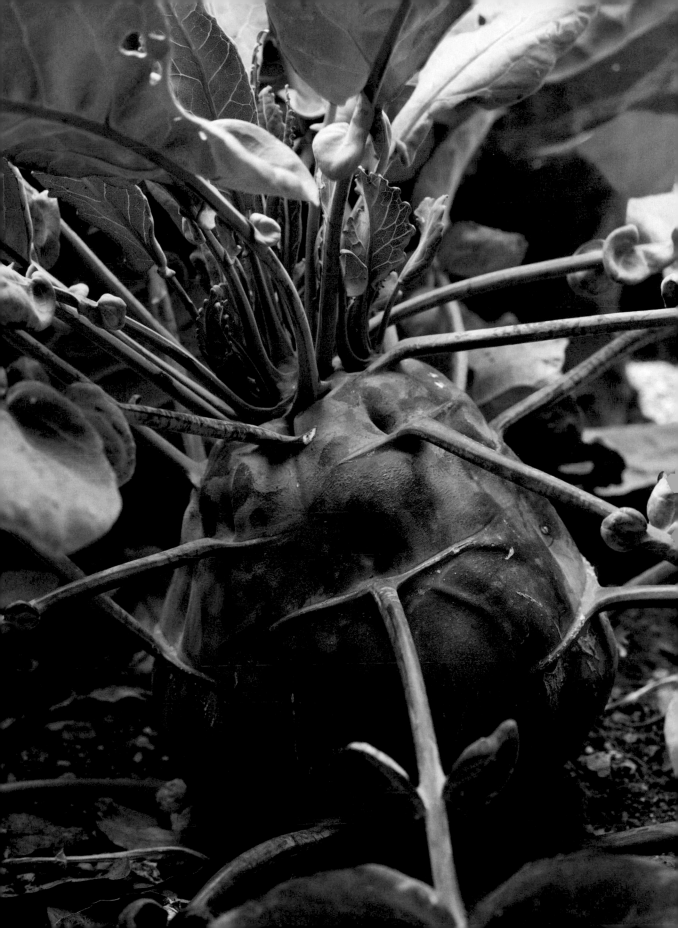

GARLIC – THE 'HEAL ALL'

Garlic, a member of the onion family, has extensive use in medicine as well as in cooking. Thought originally to come from Asia, it has a long history of use throughout the world. The Egyptians gave an allowance of garlic to their slaves to keep up their strength. Greek athletes considered that it gave them energy, and the Romans valued it greatly. The Greek physician Galen called garlic the 'heal all' and over the centuries it has been used for a variety of problems – as an antibiotic and an expectorant, and to treat thrombosis, worms, leprosy and even diabetes. In the eighteenth century, Culpeper recommended garlic to heal skin diseases and believed that there were few problems that it would not help.

The Chinese use it to treat digestive problems, whooping cough and skin diseases, and it has been shown in trials to reduce blood cholesterol levels.

In medieval Europe garlic was used as an ingredient of 'thieves' vinegar' with which thieves would protect themselves while robbing the bodies of plague victims; and it was used as an emergency antiseptic in the First World War. Its antibiotic effects are thought to be due to allicin, named from garlic's botanical name *Allium sativum*, and which is the constituent of the essential oils of garlic that give its characteristic smell.

With such a repertoire of uses, it is not surprising that it has entered folklore: garlic cloves have been carried to protect against evil (hence the origin of its common name 'devil's posy') and it was thought to be both an aphrodisiac and able to repel vampires.

Garlic in cooking

Despite its current popularity, garlic was eschewed as 'peasant's food' in Britain during the Middle Ages and was known pejoratively as 'camphor of the poor'. The French and Italians, however, have always enjoyed using garlic in their cuisines, and the French hold special feasts at the time of the garlic harvest, with every item on the menu containing it. In Gilroy, California, which supplies the USA with its garlic, there is an annual garlic festival that is celebrated with great razzmatazz.

The pervasive smell of garlic is released from the various sulphurous compounds it contains when the tissues are crushed. These odours can be absorbed by the intestine or by the skin and then exhaled or emitted from the skin. People who find garlic unpleasant can take it medicinally in capsules that are tasteless, or take it in soup in which it has been boiled to remove the smell. Raw parsley is known to reduce the smell of garlic on the breath.

The main producers of garlic are now Spain, Egypt and Argentina, though it is also a significant crop in China, Thailand, France and Italy. The best places for cultivation in Britain are the warm areas of the south coast and Isle of Wight which come closest to having the high light levels and long

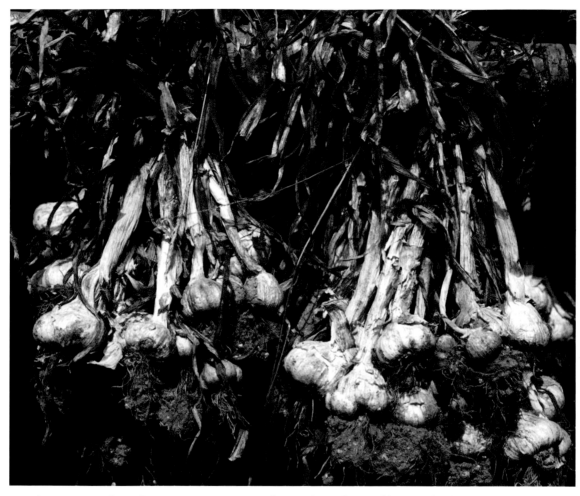

growing season of southern Europe. For people who enjoy collecting wild food and prefer mild garlic, ramsons (*Allium ursinum*) a pretty woodland species with broad leaves and white flowerheads, is common enough not to be threatened by such action. Collect this in areas that are too cool and damp to grow well-flavoured true garlic.

Growing garlic

Obtain large, firm garlic bulbs and divide them into individual cloves. Reject the small ones (use them for cooking) and plant the largest cloves 3–4cm (1½in) deep and 15cm (6in) apart in well-manured ground in full sun. Plant either in late autumn, or in early spring in areas with cold, wet winters. Keep the bed free of weeds and remove the flowerheads when they appear. Allow the crop to die down in midsummer and harvest the bulbs in late summer. Dry them off on a rack in a cool, dry, well-ventilated shed. Store them in strings (like onions), or loose in a netted bag in an airy room with a temperature under 20°C (68°F).

GARLIC BULBS HUNG UP TO DRY. GARLIC HAS A WIDE RANGE OF HEALTH APPLICATIONS IN FOLKLORE AND IN MODERN HERBAL MEDICINE.

GROWING FRUIT

Fruit is an important part of a healthy balanced diet; it helps supply vitamins, minerals, antioxidants and plenty of fibre to assist the digestive system. If you have a fairly large garden you can grow a wide variety of fruit yourself, with the advantage of knowing that your produce is free of the pesticides that commercial fruit farmers use. Even the smallest gardens usually have space for one or two fruit trees on dwarfing rootstock, or for fruit trees trained into space-saving ornamental shapes, such as espaliers and cordons.

Soft fruit

Soft fruit can be considered in three categories. Cane fruit, such as raspberries, blackberries, tayberries and loganberries, produce fruit on canes that need to be supported. Bush fruits, such as black, red and white currants, blueberries and gooseberries, grow on free-standing bushes. The third category is fruit produced on ground-hugging plants; wild and cultivated strawberries are the best examples.

If you have a professional attitude to gardening you will grow all your soft fruit in a cotton or nylon mesh fruit cage to prevent bird damage. It is always worth investing in a treated timber post and wire support for your cane fruit.

Cane fruit should be bought as dormant one- or two-year-old plants and put into well-manured soil some time in the winter when the ground is not frozen. Plant raspberries 45cm (18in) apart and the other soft fruits 2.4m (8ft) apart to allow

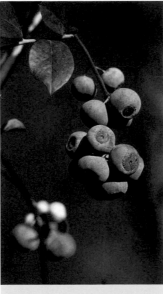

BLUEBERRIES NEED ACID SOIL TO GROW AND FRUIT WELL.

for training the canes. Most raspberries fruit on the previous year's canes, so cut the canes that have fruited down to the ground in the autumn and tie in the new growth. (The exceptions are the delicious autumn-fruiting varieties such as 'Autumn Bliss' which fruit on current growth and are pruned in winter.) Blackberries, tayberries and loganberries are pruned after fruiting; take out the old growth and tie in the new. All cane fruits are excellent for freezing.

Bush fruits should be bought as two-year-old plants and spaced 1.5m (5ft) apart. (Blueberries need acid soil and should be planted 1.2m (4ft) apart.) Again, prepare the ground well and plant during mild weather in the dormant season. Prune bush fruit during winter. Aim to take out a third of the old wood of black currants. Red and white currants and gooseberries are spur-pruned: that is, their side growth is cut back to within 7cm (2½in) of the stems. They then produce fruit on these

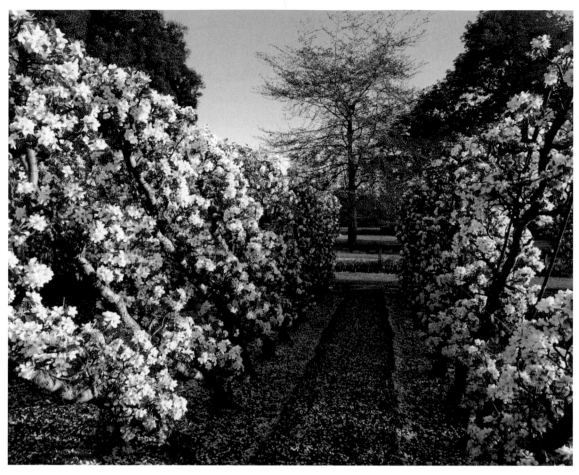

spurs. Blueberries need a proportion of the oldest shoots to be taken out in winter to keep up the vigour of the plant.

Strawberries are best planted as young pot-grown runners in late summer so that they can become established before winter. Set them 30cm (12in) apart into well-manured soil. The plants will crop well for three years, providing you remove the runners. Replace the stock after this time. Strawberries need 'strawing up' in early summer; this involves placing straw under the leaves and young fruit to keep them clean for

picking. To obtain early crops, put cloches over the plants during the winter. You can also grow strawberries in special strawberry pots; they can be successful grown this way if the soil is not allowed to dry out.

Tree fruit

You can grow quite a variety of tree or 'top' fruit in a relatively small space, providing you pay attention to training methods and getting the right rootstock. Most apples, pears, sweet cherries and some plums are not self-fertile and need

TRAINING FRUIT IN ROW CORDONS IS AN EXCELLENT WAY TO
GAIN A LARGE CROP FROM A SMALL SPACE.

to be planted close to another variety of the same fruit so that insects can cross-pollinate them. If you do have space for two varieties, plant a 'family' tree – that is one that has a number of varieties grafted on to it.

Apples and pears can be grown as free-standing trees on a rootstock chosen to produce the size of tree suitable for your garden. Alternatively they can be trained against a wall or against a post and wire fence. Cordon trees produce fruit on spurs off a single stem trained at forty-five degrees. Espalier trees fruit on spurs produced

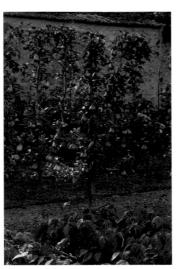

on tiers of horizontal branches. Low espaliers (with one or two tiers) make attractive divisions in the fruit garden or can be used in place of hedges.

Plums, gages and cherries can often be bought as fan-trained trees, ready to plant against a wall. The sour Morello cherry (delicious in pies) is an excellent choice for a shady wall. Apricots, peaches and nectarines are also available as fans but may be expensive. They must be planted against a very warm wall and need no pollinator varieties, but you must be prepared to train in the shoots.

RECOMMENDED VARIETIES OF FRUIT

Soft fruit		Top fruit	
Blackberries	'Bedford Giant'	Apples	'James Grieve' with 'Queen Cox'
	'Oregon Thornless' (for the patio)		or 'Ribston Pippin' with 'Egremont
Black currants	'Baldwin'		Russet'
	'Ben Lomond'	Apricots	'Moorpark'
Blueberries	'Bluecrop'		'Farmingdale'
	'Herbert'	Cherries	'Stella' (self-fertile)
Gooseberries	'White Smith'		or 'Van' with 'Merton Glory'
	'Whinham's Industry'	Gages	'Oullins Golden Gage' (self-fertile)
Loganberries	'Thornless'		'Old Greengage' (self-fertile)
	'LY 50' (a virus-free type)	Nectarines	'Elruge'
Raspberries	'Malling Jewel'		'Lord Napier'
	'Autumn Bliss'	Peaches	'Rochester'
Red currants	'Red Lake'	Pears	'Doyenne du Comice' with
Strawberries	'Royal Sovereign'		'Winter Nellis'
	(if you can obtain it virus-free)	Plums	'Coe's Golden Drop' with
White currants	'White Versailles'		'Dennison's Superb'

FORMALLY TRAINED FRUIT REPRESENTS AN INVESTMENT OF TIME AND SKILL BUT IT PAYS OFF
FOR ORNAMENT AND CAN REPLACE AN UNPRODUCTIVE FENCE.

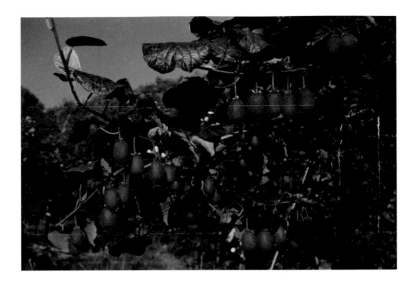

UNUSUAL FRUIT

There is a range of fruits that are simply uncommon; this is not because they are difficult to grow, though some of them do need the shelter of a warm wall, and some will only fruit well in a conservatory.

Actinidia deliciosa Chinese gooseberry
or Kiwi fruit
This delicious green fruit is healthily low in calories and extremely high in vitamin C, and is excellent as a dessert fruit, in fruit salads and pavlovas. The female vines on which it grows need pollinating by a male plant. It needs full sun, and does best in a loam-based compost in a conservatory. *Hardiness zone 7 but minimum 7°C to fruit.*

Cydonia oblonga Quince
The quince is a small tree which produces large pale pink flowers in late spring and pear-like fruit

that ripen in mid autumn. They make an excellent jam or jelly, can be candied with sugar or used to make 'quince cheese', a delicious dessert dish. Best grown on a protected wall as a fan-trained specimen. *Hardiness zone 4 but requires warmth to ripen fruit well.*

Cyphomandra crassicaulis Tamarillo
This is sometimes called the tree tomato because it produces fruits somewhat like an oval plum tomato, though they are sharper in taste. Its fruits are good in tarts and are high in vitamin C. It is best grown in a loam-based compost in a conservatory or glasshouse border. *Hardiness zone 9, but minimum 12°C to fruit.*

Diospyros kaki Persimmon or Sharon fruit
This fruit is native to China and Japan and will only bear fruit in a warm climate such as the Mediterranean area, Australia or the southern

KIWI FRUIT (*ACTINIDIA DELICIOSA*) WILL FRUIT IN THREE YEARS FROM
PLANTING IF A MALE VINE IS NEARBY.

USA. It is a tall tree and produces orange, astringent fruits reminiscent of a tomato. Female cultivars need pollinating by a male cultivar. They are delicious candied. *Hardiness zone 8.*

Eriobotrya japonica Loquat

This is an elegant small tree or large shrub that needs a sheltered sunny spot to produce the yellow fruits that appear in the spring, following an autumn flowering. Native to China and Japan, it is widely planted throughout the Mediterranean region. It needs fertile, well-drained soil and protection from wind. Eat loquats in pies; they are a good source of vitamins. *Hardiness zone 7.*

Ficus carica Fig

Figs need a very warm and sheltered spot, preferably on a sunny wall, and the fruit ripens best after a long, hot summer. Constrict their roots in a brick-built box 60cm (2ft) square by as much deep, sunken into the ground at the foot of the wall. This will encourage fruit at the expense of leaf growth. The variety 'Brown Turkey' is a classic. Figs are a gentle laxative. *Hardiness zone 7.*

Mespilus germanica Medlar

The medlar is a small tree that flowers in early summer. It needs subtropical conditions for the curious brown fruits to ripen fully, but in cooler climates the fruits are picked in late autumn and allowed to become almost rotten before eating. This 'bletted' fruit is then enjoyed as a delicacy with port or madeira. It has a granular texture and, to my mind, tastes like a rich pear. Plant a named variety, such as 'Nottingham' or 'Dutch',

in a sunny position in a well-drained soil. *Hardiness zone 8.*

Morus nigra Mulberry

Because the fruit must be fully ripe when picked and will not stand market handling, mulberries are almost never available commercially. A mulberry tree will produce fruit when quite young and trees live to a great age. A tip when the tree is of a good size is to naturalize bulbs under it and not mow under it until midsummer. This means that when the fruit matures in late summer and some inevitably drop it will not mark a prized lawn. Mulberries make excellent jam and wine, and are delicious with ice cream and in summer puddings. *Hardiness zone 5.*

Physalis peruviana Cape gooseberry

Once cultivated around the Cape of Good Hope, this perennial plant produces a slightly acid, bright yellow berry with an inflated calyx. The berries make curious novelties as dessert fruit, and are easy to grow in any soil in slight shade. *Hardiness zone 8.*

Punica granatum Pomegranate

This Asian tree is now naturalized throughout the subtropics, and fruits well in a Mediterranean climate. In cooler places, pomegranates can be successfully grown as standard trees in tubs, treated like citrus and given protection in the winter under glass. Flowers and fruit are carried on current year's growth. They have an acid, seedy pulp rather like a passion fruit, and are quite a good laxative. *Hardiness zone 9.*

HOW TO GROW TROPICAL FRUIT PLANTS FROM PIPS

Many attractive plants can be grown easily from the pips of tropical fruits. All you need is a simple electric propagator to provide a good temperature, a good compost and enough light when the seeds have germinated.

This is a hobby that adults and children alike find fascinating. How delightful to have your own miniature fruit orchard! Here are some suggestions of fruits easily available in supermarkets.

Fruit	Botanical name	Germination method	Temperature	Compost
Avocado	*Persea americana*	Part submerge in water with the pointed end uppermost. Pot on when shoot/root is well emerged.	18°C (65°F) (ambient room temperature)	
Cherimoya	*Annona cherimola*	Plant in compost, with the seed just covered.	21°C (70°F)	John Innes No.2
Christophine	*Sechium edule*	Plant the large single seed part-covered by compost.	16°C (60°F)	John Innes No.2
Date*	*Phoenix dactylifera*	Place in moist vermiculite in a polythene bag in a propagator or airing cupboard. Pot each one up once a root has emerged.	21°C (70°F)	John Innes No.1
Grapefruit	*Citrus × paradisi*	Sow fresh seeds from really ripe fruit. Plant shallowly.	16–21°C (60–70°F)	John Innes Seed Compost
Guava	*Psidium guajava*	Sow fresh seed.	16–21°C (60–70°F)	John Innes Seed Compost
Kumquat	*Fortunella* spp.	As for grapefruit.	16°C (60°F)	John Innes Seed Compost
Loquat	*Eriobotrya japonica*	As for grapefruit.	13°C (55°F)	John Innes Seed Compost
Mango*	*Mangifera indica*	Plant the flattened stone sharp edge down.	21–24°C (70–75°F)	John Innes No.2
Passion fruit	*Passiflora edulis*	Sow fresh seed in its pulp.	18°C (65°F)	John Innes No.2
Pawpaw	*Carica papaya*	Sow fresh seed.	18°C (65°F)	John Innes No.2
Pomegranate	*Punica granatum*	Sow fresh or dried seed in spring.	21°C (70°F)	John Innes Seed Compost
Rambutan	*Nephelium lappaceum*	Sow fresh seed.	21–24°C (70–75°F)	John Innes Seed Compost
Starfruit	*Averrhoa carambola*	Sow fresh seed.	21°C (70°F)	John Innes Seed Compost

* Cover seed with very hot (not boiling) water and leave to soak for twenty-four hours before sowing.

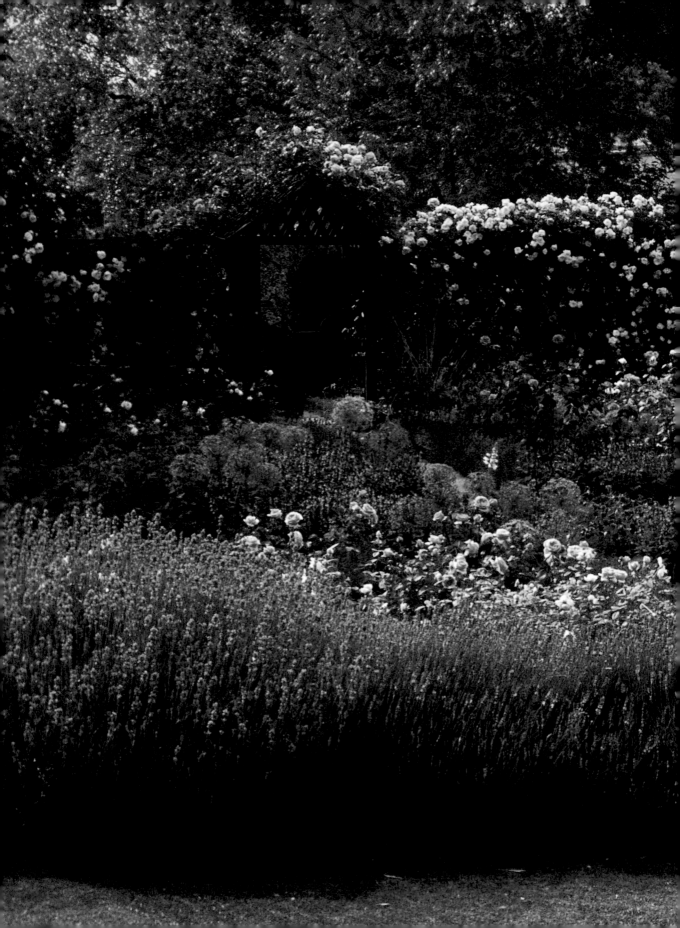

AWAKENING THE
SENSES

PLANTS GIVE US PLEASURE AND CAN BRING HEALING THROUGH OUR FIVE SENSES — TASTE, SIGHT, HEARING, SMELL AND TOUCH — EITHER PHYSICALLY or more indirectly via memories and moods. Herbs can enhance your enjoyment of, and delight in, the taste of good food; the pleasures are multiplied if the herbs are home-grown. The look of a garden depends largely on its colours and shapes, and our choice of plants and the way we put them together is limited only by imagination. Colour is one of the most potent means of evoking mood and atmosphere in a garden; but it needs skill and patience to be successful, especially as it involves the fourth dimension, time. Therapeutic sounds can also be introduced into a garden – the trickle of water, the swish of a bamboo, the buzz of a bee – and these can also affect mood beneficially. The evocative power of scent is perhaps even more invigorating: it can stimulate memory and be used to evoke happy times to heal us psychologically. Then there are plants which are a joy to touch, whose texture can surprise and delight us. With thought and planning, our gardens can awake our senses.

TONING COLOURS CREATE A HARMONIOUS EFFECT FOR THE EYE IN THIS GARDEN BUT
TOUCHING THESE PLANTS WILL RELEASE SCENT TOO.

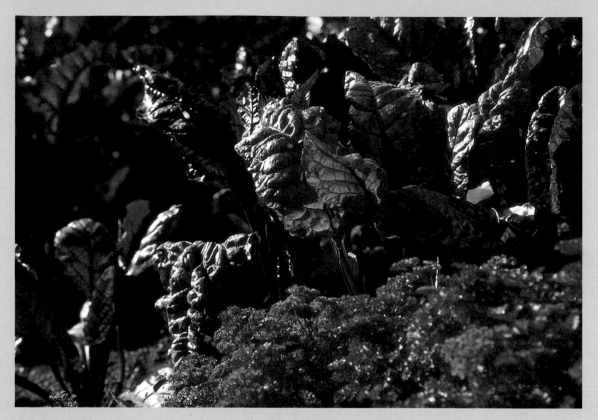

TASTE
PLEASING THE PALATE

Herbs are used in cookery to bring out and emphasize the natural flavours of foods or to complement them. Sometimes herbs are used to aid digestion; the slightly bitter taste of sage, for example, stimulates the flow of bile which helps to digest fat, and one of the properties of mint is to calm the digestive tract. Herbs also make attractive garnishes, adding visual enjoyment to the dish. It is possible to preserve some herbs, by drying, freezing or salting them, but nothing quite competes with the taste of freshly picked herbs, so it is always worth growing your own even if you then preserve the surplus. And in the same way that herbs make attractive gar-nishes, they also make attractive gardens in their own right. Most of the plants take little space, so even urban gardeners can find ways of having their own small herb garden, whether simply in a window box or in a small bed close to the house.

PARSLEY IS A TRADITIONAL GARNISH HERB. THE PALATE IS ALSO TEASED BY VISUAL RICHNESS
ON THE PLATE – AS WITH THIS RUBY CHARD.

THE MAINSTAY CULINARY HERBS

By tradition, certain herbs are used with certain dishes, and some are strongly linked with national or regional cuisines. If you try using them in unconventional ways, or using those that are less run-of-the-mill, you may reawaken your taste buds.

Allium schoenoprasum Chives

This clump-forming, bulbous perennial grows to 20–30 × 20–30cm (8–12 × 8–12in) and produces pale purple to pink flowers in the summer. The leaves are used in salads, omelettes and soups, and blended with sour cream as a topping. Sow seeds in spring, and propagate thereafter by division in spring every few years. *Hardiness zone 5.*

Aloysia triphylla Lemon verbena

This deciduous shrub, reaching 3 × 2m (9 × 6ft), is often trained onto a wall. Its lemon-scented leaves are used in fruit salads, fruit drinks or punch, and can also be used to flavour custards, ice cream and sorbets. Plant out after all danger of frost is past, in full sun at the foot of a sheltered wall, and protect from frost in winter. Take cuttings in early summer for further stock. *Hardiness zone 8.*

Anethum graveolens Dill

An annual with feathery aromatic foliage, dill grows to 60 × 23cm (24 × 9in). The leaves can be chopped into fish sauces and into salads; and the seed is commonly used in the pickling of cucum-

CHIVES ARE A TROUBLE-FREE HERB GROWN FOR THEIR LEAVES BUT ORNAMENTAL IN FLOWER. THEY PREFER WELL-DRAINED SOIL.

ber and gherkins. Sow seed successionally throughout the spring and early summer. Dill needs to grow in rich, moist soil in sun to reach its full potential and may bolt in dry weather. *Hardiness zone 8.*

Angelica archangelica Angelica

This stately biennial or mono-carpic herb grows to 2m × 60cm (6 × 2ft) and produces rounded heads of tiny chartreuse-green flowers in early summer. The young stems can be candied to decorate cakes by cooking with sugar or honey. It is best in slight shade in moist soil. Sow seed in late summer, and thin seedlings to 30cm (12in) apart. *Hardiness zone 4.*

Anthriscus cereifolium Chervil

Grown as an annual, this herb grows to 60 × 30cm (2 × 1ft) and has bright green, finely divided foliage. The leaves are used in salads, soups and sauces, and are traditionally used in egg dishes and as a vegetable garnish. Sow successionally throughout the spring and early summer in well-drained soil in partial shade. Hot, dry summers will cause it to bolt. *Hardiness zone 7.*

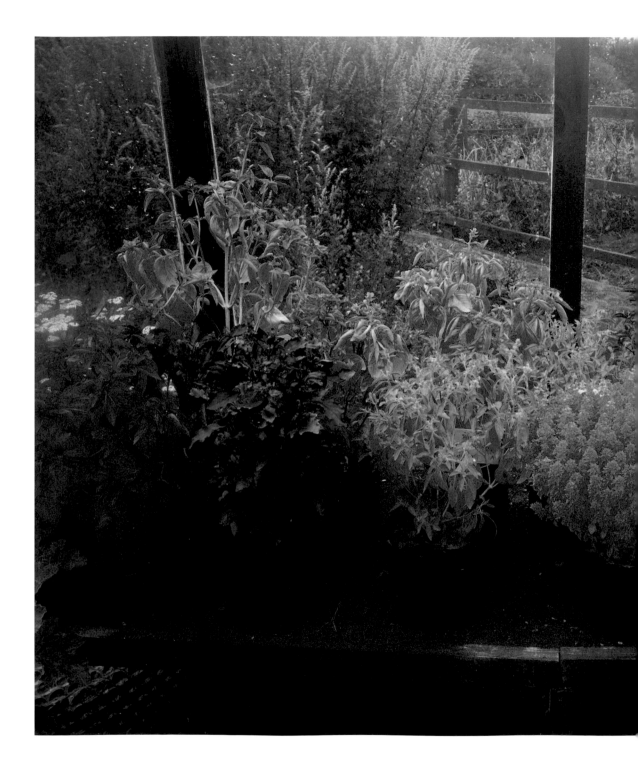

A COLLECTION OF BASILS, INCLUDING PURPLE-LEAVED FORMS. ALL BASILS ARE EXTREMELY FROST-SENSITIVE, SO BRING THEM UNDER COVER AS THE SEASON MATURES.

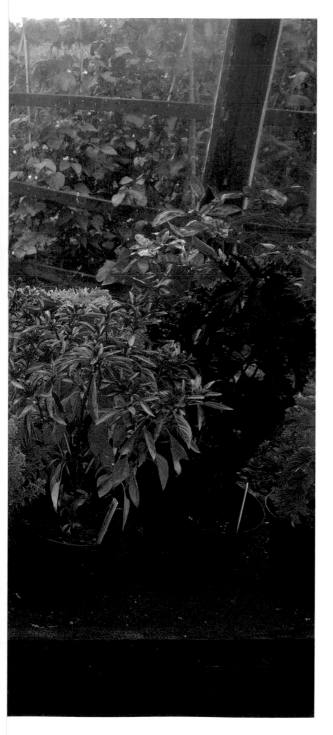

and are invasive, so grow them in an isolated patch, or in a sunken tub (with the bottom removed).

Monarda didyma Bergamot, or Bee balm

This perennial grows to 120 × 60cm (4 × 2ft) and has scarlet flowers in summer. The fragrance resembles the bergamot oil that is used to flavour Earl Grey tea. Bergamot leaves and flowers can be added to green salads, fruit salads, fruit cups and jellies. Plant in rich soil in light shade (it is subject to powdery mildew in dry conditions). Increase by division in spring or autumn. *Hardiness zone 4.*

Myrrhis odorata Sweet cicely

This perennial grows to 120 × 90cm (4 × 3ft) and has fern-like, anise-scented foliage. The leaves can be used to sweeten tart fruit during cooking as an alternative to cane or beet sugar, or added to omelettes, salads and fruit salads. Sow in the open ground in spring, in moist soil and partial shade. *Hardiness zone 5.*

Ocimum basilicum Basil, or Sweet basil and *Ocimum basilicum* 'Minimum' Bush basil

Both types of basil are annual; sweet basil grows to 20–60 × 30cm (8–24 × 12in), and bush basil to 15–30 × 15cm (6–12 × 6in), and both are grown and used in the same way. Basil is the finest herb for use in Mediterranean dishes, especially with tomatoes. Sow the seeds under glass in mid spring and do not plant out until all risk of frost is past. Basil does best in a sheltered, warm spot, in well-drained compost. *Hardiness zone 10.*

PRESERVING AND STORING HERBS

A good crop of herbs can be preserved for use during the winter by drying, freezing or salting down. It is certainly worth doing this for any of the Mediterranean herbs, which really need the summer's heat to produce their full flavour and languish if grown in pots on the window sill in winter in a misguided attempt to prolong summer's yield.

Drying

The herbs that dry best are thyme, rosemary, bay, marjoram and sage. Pick herbs on a dry morning when the dew has evaporated, and choose growth that is in bud but has not yet produced flowers. You can dry the sprigs in several ways. Either hang them up to dry in a warm, airy place out of direct sunlight, or lay them on a tray covered with muslin and put them in a warm place, such as the warming drawer of an oven, or an airing cupboard, for a few days until they are dry but retain their greenness. Do not leave sprigs of herbs hanging up for any length of time; they may look decorative but the herbs will dry to a dusty, tasteless condition if their flavour is not sealed.

When the herbs are dry, either wrap them whole in paper or, to save space, crumble them, discarding the woodier stems, and bottle them. Whether whole or crumbled, all herbs should be stored in a dry, dark place, as light will destroy their flavour.

Freezing

Another way to preserve herbs is to freeze them.

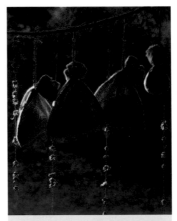

A TRADITIONAL DUTCH WAY OF AIR-DRYING HERBS. THEN STORE THEM IN A DARK, DRY PLACE.

This is a particularly good method for tender-leaved herbs, such as basil, parsley, fennel and dill, which do not dry well, and for sprigs of tarragon. When freezing large-leaved basil, pick individual leaves and freeze them in small freezer bags. If you have a large ice-making compartment you can produce a supply of herb ice cubes, ready for soups, sauces or stews, by chopping the herbs, adding a little water and freezing the mixtures. Remember to label the ice cube trays. For grilled meat and fish, you can mix the herbs in butter and then freeze the mixture to add to a grill when needed.

Salting

Basil leaves are rather fleshy and do not dry well, and if you do not want to freeze them, you can preserve them by salting them. Add salt between layers of leaves and then cover with olive or grapeseed oil. This will preserve basil for up to four weeks and when mixed with vinegar, garlic and black pepper will make a good vinaigrette dressing – especially for that wonderful appetizer, tomato and mozzarella cheese.

LOVAGE LEAVES (OPPOSITE, FOREGROUND) CAN BE DRIED
TO MAKE A SWEET AND FRAGRANT HERBAL TEA.

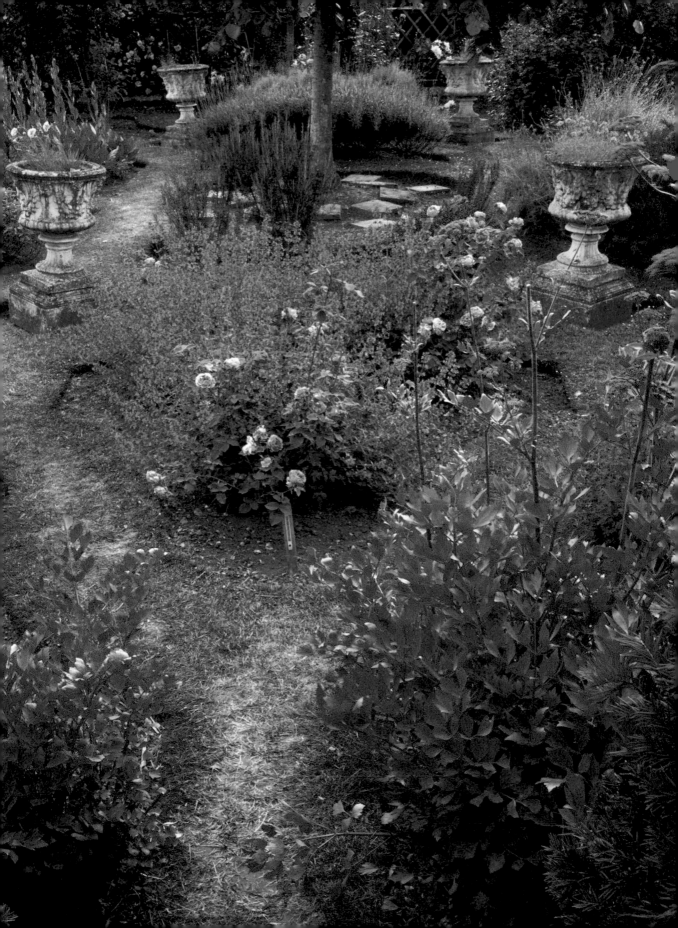

SIGHT
PLANNING A PLEASING OUTLOOK

Many of the key elements of a garden – its overall design, the shapes and colours of its planting – are visually perceived, and whatever your taste in garden style, a garden that satisfies your eye will also engender a strong sense of psychological well-being.

Landscape architects and garden designers frequently talk of the 'bones' of a garden, by which they mean the permanent features, such as walls, terraces, paths and pergolas, that define the basic layout and provide a framework for the plants. Getting the structure right so that it brings you visual pleasure is as important as the planting. (See pages 152–4 for advice on garden design.)

The visual pleasure that you get from the planting in your garden will come as much from the shapes of the plants, and how they are grouped together, as it will from the colours. The effect of the shapes of plants is sometimes called 'form' in garden design: that is, the overall combination of spiky, rounded, conical and feathery outlines that give three-dimensional shape to a planting. You can choose from a wide variety of trees, shrubs and perennials that can be combined and contrasted to give a pleasing balance of soft, hard-edged and spiky plants.

Some species fulfil several patterns in that they have large hard-edged leaves and delicate masses of feathery flowers; for example, *Crambe*

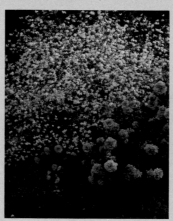

CRAMBE CORDIFOLIA HAS DELIGHTFULLY FEATHERY FLOWERS CREATING A DIFFUSE AND AIRY EFFECT..

cordifolia and *Crambe maritima*. Here the fourth dimension in garden design is introduced, that of time. The effect that a plant gives may well depend on its growth stage at a particular time of year. For example, the crambe has clearly defined edges in spring but is soft when covered with profuse panicles of flowers in early summer. Many conifers look hard in outline except in early spring when their soft new growth appears.

Some unusually shaped plants can be used almost as sculptures in the garden. The monkey puzzle (*Araucaria araucana*) is a good candidate for this sort of treatment. Plants with strong leaves are usually best placed against a hard landscaped background for their form to be enjoyed.

Among the most useful plants for structural effect are ferns and grasses. Fern leaves are not always 'ferny' – some (for example *Asplenium scolopendrium*) are strongly strap-shaped – but generally they soften plantings in the summer months. Grasses provide vertical accent and do it softly. In winter they also provide a skeleton for the 'rime' of hoar frosts.

THE RIME OF WINTER FROST ACCENTUATES EVERY NEEDLE ON THESE CONIFERS (OPPOSITE).
THIS IS A VISUAL PLEASURE ONLY – WALKING ON THE GRASS WILL KILL IT.

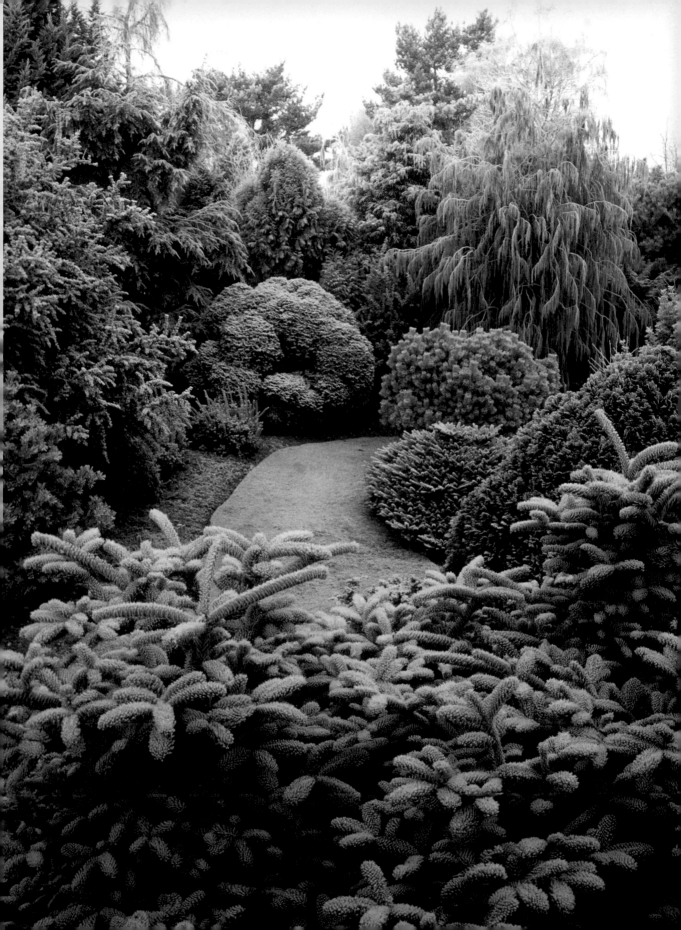

THE POWER OF COLOUR

The pleasure given by colour is one of the blessings of sight. This is as true of designing with colourful plants as it is in art, and perhaps it is no coincidence that many of the ideas about plant colour groupings come via gardeners trained in art or photography.

In the nineteenth century the English painter J.M.W. Turner used colour in his work to portray light and atmosphere, banishing the conventional use of greyish foregrounds and green mid-distance pigments in favour of reds in the foreground, yellow in the mid-distance and white or blue in the far distance. Gertrude Jekyll, the great Victorian gardener, would certainly have known of Turner's lectures at the Royal Academy in London and his influence is noticeable in some of her border designs. A direct line of her ideas can be traced, through her book *Colour in the Flower Garden* (1908), to some of the finest English gardens: Sissinghurst in Kent, Hidcote Manor in Gloucestershire, Tintinhull in Somerset and Great Dixter in Sussex, among others. The rose garden of Dumbarton Oaks, near Washington, DC, shows her influence, and her theories are also popular in many private gardens in New Zealand. You can gain many ideas from visiting these gardens and you may find that your ideas on colour evolve, even from the belief that no colours clash in nature.

In the past few decades much attention has been paid by interior designers to the way that colour in the home can affect mood and express personality. Since Penelope Hobhouse, in her book *Colour in Your Garden* (1985), made a radical advance on Gertrude Jekyll's theories of colour in the garden, there has been a revival of interest in colour associations between plants as outdoor design features. The concept of colour as 'healing' – in the sense of being designed to ameliorate mood – in the garden is the logical extension of the use of colour in interior design, especially in the perception of town or courtyard gardens as being 'outdoor rooms', an extension of living space. It is possible to design both foliage and flower colour in your garden to create effects to match or to change your mood. On pages 105–7 there are some suggestions, colour by colour, for you to consider.

People vary greatly in their colour preferences. We all have different psychological, emotional and physical responses to colour, and everyone's 'eye' is different. The basic principles of the artist's 'colour wheel', however, and the theories that underlie it can help you plan the

BEING SEATED AMONG SUCH HOT COLOURS IS UNLIKELY TO BE CALMING – BUT IT MAY WELL CHEER YOUR SPIRITS.

MIXING PINK WITH YELLOW (OPPOSITE) WAS ONCE A FAUX PAS BUT HAS NOW BECOME FASHIONABLE. YOUR TASTE SHOULD BE PARAMOUNT.

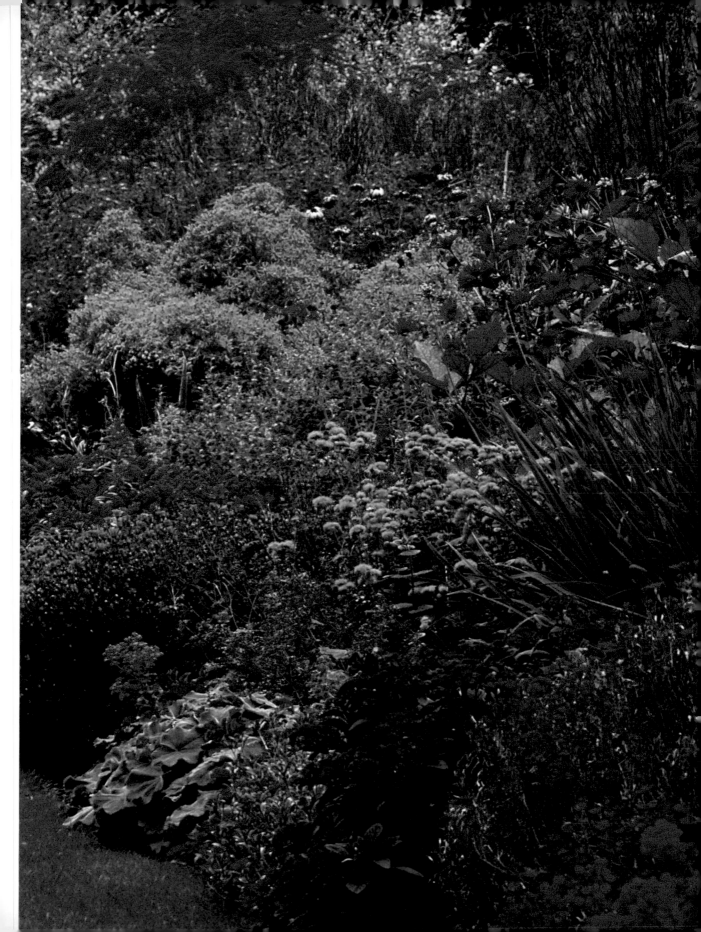

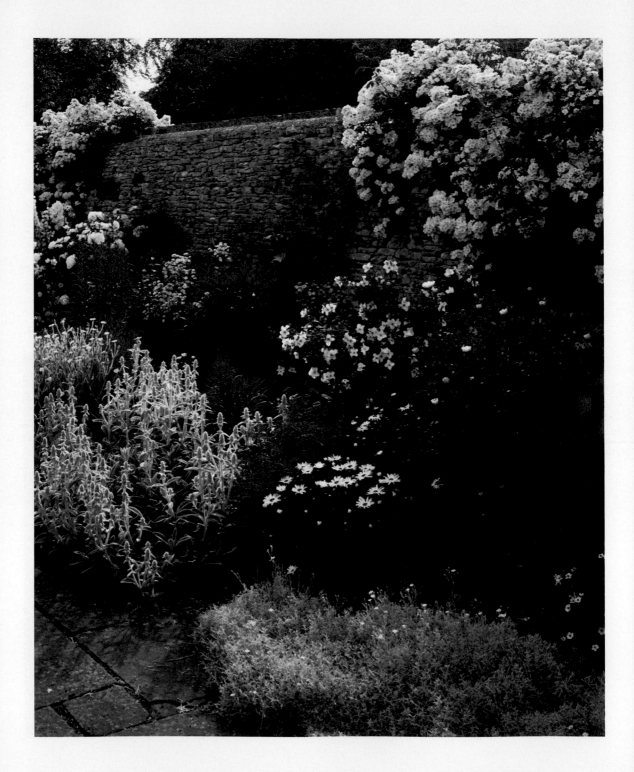

WHITE GARDENS EXCEL IN EVENING LIGHT. REMEMBER TO DESIGN THEM IN
THREE DIMENSIONS, USING ANY AVAILABLE WALLS OR FENCES.

A WHITE PLANTING TO BE ENJOYED IN EARLY SUMMER

Start by plotting the structure: trees and most significant shrubs. Then fill in with perennials in groups of three or five. Plant bulbs between and among them. Use climbers on tripods for vertical accent if your area does not include walls. Finally, plant annuals in pots or tubs, or in any gaps in front of your composition.

Botanical name	Maximum height & spread	Comment
TREES		
Halesia caroliniana	7.5 × 7.5m (25 × 25ft)	Best tree for the average-sized garden.
Styrax japonica	6 × 6m (20 × 20ft)	Best tree for the small-sized garden.
PERENNIALS		
Campanula alliariifolia 'Ivory Bells'	60 × 45cm (2 × 1½ft)	Very elegant pendant flowers.
Crambe cordifolia	1.8 × 1.2m (6 × 4ft)	Creates a haze of white flowers.
Dianthus 'Mrs Sinkins'	30 × 30–45cm (12 × 12–18in)	For a dry, sunny spot. Good on chalk soils.
Dicentra eximia 'Alba'	30–45 × 30cm (12–18 × 12in)	Needs moisture.
Digitalis purpurea – white strains	1.2 × 0.3m (4 × 1ft)	Best in semi-shade.
Hesperis matronalis 'Alba'	1 × 0.6m (3 × 2ft)	Lovely at night, when it is also scented.
Papaver orientale 'Black and White'	60 × 60cm (2 × 2ft)	Needs full sun.
Zantedeschia aethiopica	90 × 60cm (3 × 2ft)	Needs moist soil and light shade.
SHRUBS		
Carpentaria californica	1.8 × 1.8m (6 × 6ft)	Only for warm gardens.
Cistus laurifolius	1.8 × 1.8m (6 × 6ft)	One of the hardiest of the cistus.
Convolvulus cneorum	1 × 1m (3 × 3ft)	Must have full sun.
Cornus kousa 'Chinensis'	4 × 3m (13 × 10ft)	Needs acid soil.
Philadelphus species, hybrids and cultivars	up to 3 × 2.5m (10 × 8ft)	Lovely, but short flowering season.
Pittosporum tobira	1–1.2 × 1m (3–4 × 3ft)	Flowers scented of orange blossom.
Syringa 'Madame Lemoine'	3.5 × 3m (12 × 10ft)	Lovely, but short flowering season.
Viburnum plicatum 'Lanarth'	3 × 3m (10 × 10ft)	Best in moist soil and light shade.
BULBS		
Camassia leichtlinii (white form)	1.2 × 0.3m (4 × 1ft)	Needs a warm position.
Convallaria majalis	20 × 30cm (8 × 12in)	Spreads if it is happy.
Lilium regale	1.2 × 0.3m (4 × 1ft)	One of the best lilies for style and scent.
ANNUALS		
Argemone grandiflora	90 × 30cm (3 × 1ft)	Delicate flowers.
Lavatera 'Mont Blanc'	60 × 30cm (2 × 1ft)	Icy white petals.
Nicotiana alata	90 × 30cm (3 × 1ft)	Flowers open in the evening.
CLIMBERS		
Jasminum officinale	9 × 4m (30 × 15ft)	Requires training, will not self-cling.
Wisteria sinensis 'Alba'	20 × 20m (65 × 65ft)	Requires spur-pruning in winter.

COMPLEMENTARY BLUES AND YELLOWS

'Colours appear what they are not, according to the ground which surrounds them,' wrote Leonardo da Vinci, an idea taken up three centuries later in the 1880s by the French Impressionist painters. They understood that one of the effects of pairs of complementary colours, such as blue with orange, violet with yellow, and red with green, is that each colour physically induces an after-image of its partner in the eye, even when the eye is closed.

This simple fact can be exploited by garden designers to intensify colour by preparing the eye in advance. For example, an area of gold foliage preceding a block of violet-blue planting will enhance that planting by its after-image effect. The eye yearns for the colour's complement and then is satisfied by it. As Gertrude Jekyll wrote, 'Now the eye has again become saturated, and has therefore by the law of complementary colour, acquired a strong appetite for the greys and purples. These therefore assume an appearance of brilliancy that they would not have had without the preparation provided by their recently received complementary colour.'

One way of using complementary colours is to design single-colour gardens that lead into one another but are physically separated by hedges. Thus a yellow garden would be followed by a blue or purple garden, or vice versa. The eye is then successively prepared and refreshed as the observer moves around the garden.

In a border where you wish to use blue and yellow try grading the blues from one end of the border to the other, using yellows as groupings within this to produce a rich and unified visual effect. Arrange the various tones of blue carefully, say with the pale and mid-blues interspersed with the gold or orange-yellows and the violet-blues with the paler yellows. This is quite a feat of planting design and is complicated by the fact that blues will often be deeper in alkaline soils.

I would also avoid using gold-foliaged plants except for spring borders, because the colour often fades as the sun becomes higher in the sky towards midsummer and the foliage may burn in a border fully exposed to the sunshine that most border plants require. Plan your border against a good green hedge as a background or against an orangey brick wall – blues and yellows look far less stunning against a fence.

Use the table on the following pages to design groups within your border – for spring, for summer or for autumn effect. Some of the suggested spring groupings, including bluebells mixed with the lime green of *Smyrnium perfoliatum*, have been used at the Royal Botanic Gardens, Kew, where an adventurous use of colour with perennial plants has been present for the past fifty years. Other gardens where colour effects are well used include Clare College gardens in Cambridge, Great Dixter in Sussex, Hadspen in Somerset (designed and run by the 'colourists' Sandra and Nori Pope), Villandry in the French Loire Valley, Versailles outside Paris and the Botanic Gardens in Auckland, New Zealand.

A MASTERLY COLOUR DESIGN IN BLUE AND YELLOW AT CLARE COLLEGE, CAMBRIDGE.

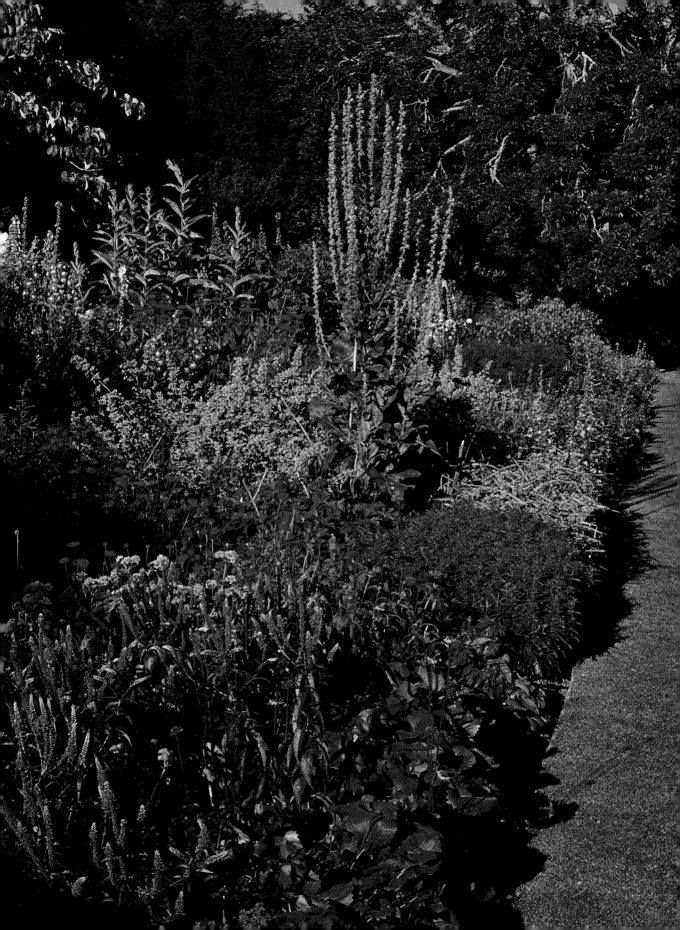

HEARING

MAKING THE MOST OF HEALING SOUNDS

Your garden can become a refuge from the noise pollution of the urban and worka-day world and the disturbance and stresses that unwanted noise produces. From the sighing and rustling of leaves and stems in the breeze to the tinkling or rushing of water, sounds in the garden can generate and influence many different moods and feelings. Sounds, like scent, can trigger vivid memories and can bring to mind happy incidents in the past, often from childhood. These can have a psychologically healing effect, especially against depression and as an antidote to the strains of everyday pressures and uncertainties.

Refreshing sounds can be produced by the movement of the wind through trees and shrubs, and there are many species you can plant for this purpose. Bamboos and grasses give gentle rustling sounds that can provide a pleasing background to more immediate sounds.

Waterfalls and fountains, producing a trickle or cascade, can be 'tuned' through careful arrangement of the height, angle and interruption of the fall of water to make 'scales' of sound, bringing an added dimension of harmony to a garden. Further ideas about the use of running water to provide refreshing sounds are given on pages 120–1.

Choosing plants that create sounds is a start, but there are also many other species that attract sounds to them. Plants and flowers that are irresistible to insects will result in a glorious drowsy hum on a sunny summer's afternoon as bees and

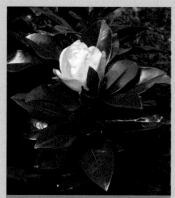

MAGNOLIA GRANDIFLORA HAS HUGE, LEMON-SCENTED FLOWERS BUT ITS LEAVES ALSO CLATTER IN THE BREEZE.

others busy themselves among the blooms. You can deliberately attract bees by specifically selecting species they use as sources of nectar or pollen. Some of the best to plant are any of the varieties of thyme, lavender and rosemary, *Phlomis*, *Lythrum*, *Eryngium*, *Cytisus*, *Verbena* and particularly *Cistus*, which also provide scent and colour in the garden.

At the Chelsea Physic Garden, where bees are kept, large numbers have been recorded on *Rosa pimpinellifolia*, *Mirabilis jalapa*, the fuller's teasel (*Dipsacus fullonum*), many of the paeonies and all of the Californian lilacs (*Ceanothus* species and varieties). You can encourage birds into the garden so that their song can be enjoyed by providing bird tables and nest boxes and also by providing the type of plants that form their natural food sources (see page 167). Further ways to attract other wildlife to the garden are suggested on pages 162–6.

THE BUZZ OF HONEY BEES (OPPOSITE) IS STRONGLY ASSOCIATED WITH HIGH SUMMER AND ITS PLEASURES.

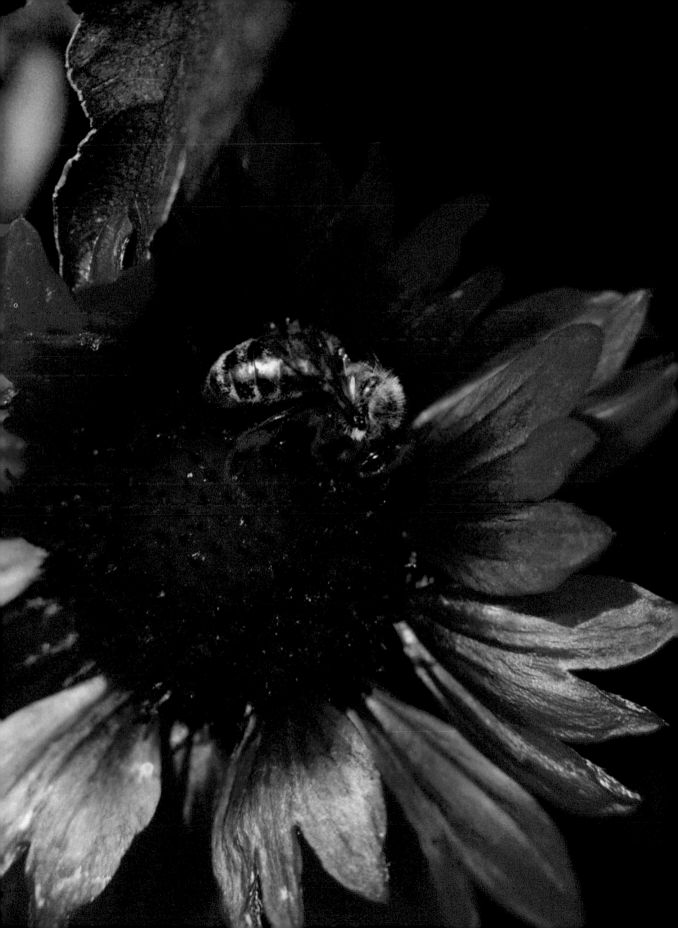

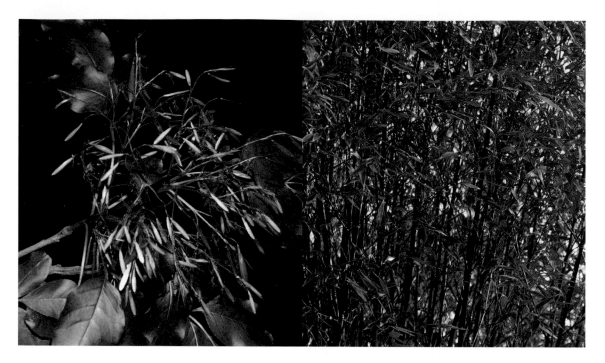

TREES, SHRUBS AND GRASSES TO PLEASE THE EAR

Betula papyrifera Paper birch
This is a light-textured deciduous tree growing to 9 × 4.5m (30 × 15ft), suitable for light, acid soils. The 'twigginess' of birches can produce attractive sounds in windy gardens. *Hardiness zone 2.*

Colutea arborescens Bladder senna
A deciduous shrub for full sun and light soil, growing to 1.8 × 2.5m (6 × 8ft), bladder senna produces inflated seed pods which rattle and rustle in the breeze and are highly attractive to children – to pop them. *Hardiness zone 5.*

Cordyline australis Cabbage palm
These evergreens are not true palms but are related to lilies and have the characteristic strap-like leaves. They eventually develop branched stems to 3.5 × 2.5m (12 × 8ft). They are good by the sea in warm areas where they rustle in the breeze. *Hardiness zone 10.*

Eucalyptus Gum tree
These evergreen trees with grey-green foliage are variable in height – most reach at least 9 × 4.5m (30 × 15ft). They are drought-tolerant, grow fast in congenial positions, and drop leaf litter which makes a crunching sound and releases the familiar aroma underfoot. *Hardiness zones 8–10.*

Ficus carica Fig
Deciduous trees that grow to 4.5 × 3.5m (15 × 12ft), figs produce huge leaves which rustle if

THE MANNA ASH (LEFT) AND THE BLACK (STEMMED) BAMBOO (RIGHT) ARE BOTH USEFUL
FOR THE RUSTLING SOUND A BREEZE PRODUCES IN THEM.

caught by a strong breeze. In climates cooler than that of their native Mediterranean they are best trained against a warm wall. *Hardiness zone 7.*

Fraxinus ornus Manna ash

This is a densely foliaged, deciduous tree with good potential to catch the wind in its crown to attractive effect. It will grow to 6 × 6m (20 × 20ft), so it is not for a small garden. Attractive autumn colour is a bonus. *Hardiness zone 6.*

Magnolia grandiflora

The bull bay magnolia from the southern states of America has extremely handsome, dark glossy green evergreen leaves which clatter together in the breeze (as well as huge, lemon-scented flowers). It will grow to 7.5 × 4.5m (20 × 15ft) and can be trained against a wall. *Hardiness zone 6.*

Miscanthus

The perennial grasses of this genus are useful for producing a gentle rustling sound. They are variable in height from 2–3 × 1m (3–9 × 3ft), the tallest species being *M. sacchariflorus*, which is almost like sugar cane and is useful as a screen. Cut the old growth down in spring and it will shoot again to 3m (9ft) in a season. *Hardiness zones 4–8.*

Phyllostachys nigra Black bamboo

Named after its stems, which darken as they age, this bamboo produces attractive rustling sounds with wind in the foliage. Like many bamboos, it spreads if it is not restricted, growing to 3–6 × 6m (10–20 × 20ft). *Hardiness zone 7.*

Phyllostachys viridi-glaucescens

This is a grey-green-stemmed bamboo that grows to 4.5–6 × 6m (15–20 × 20ft), so it is best in an unrestricted space. The heavy canes of mature clumps will 'creak' with friction. *Hardiness zone 7.*

Picea breweriana

Brewer's weeping spruce

A small coniferous tree, growing to 6 × 2.5m (12 × 8ft), it is charming for its spreading, dipping branches and for the characteristic sound of the breeze in conifers. *Hardiness zone 6.*

Pinus bungeana Lacebark pine

Growing to 3.5 × 1.5m (12 × 5ft), this is one of the best pines for small gardens. It is useful for the sound of the breeze through its pine foliage as well as its pretty bark. *Hardiness zone 5.*

Populus tremula Aspen tree and
Populus tremuloides American aspen

These deciduous trees with rather pendant foliage are well-known for the 'tremulous' sound produced by the wind through their branches. *P. tremula* is suitable only for large gardens or as a boundary tree because it will grow to 12 × 9m (40 × 30ft). *P. tremuloides* is more modest at 6–9 × 4.5m (20–30ft × 15ft). *Hardiness zones 2 and 1, respectively.*

Sinarundinaria nitida

This is an evergreen, clump-forming (rather than invasive) bamboo, well suited to the smaller garden where rustling sound is desired. It will grow to 2.5–4 × 2m (8–13 × 7ft). *Hardiness zone 5.*

SMELL
HARNESSING THE POWER OF SCENT

Perfumed plants in the garden have a particular charm whether their fragrance is emitted from flowers or through crushing the foliage. Our appreciation of fragrance is, of course, incidental to the reason why plants produce scented essential oils. In the case of flowers this is nearly always to attract pollinators.

Night-scented flowers are coloured specifically to attract night-flying insects and moths: they are mostly white, cream or very pale yellow to show up in the dark, with tubular flowers adapted to long-tongued pollinators searching for nectar, and their perfume is given off only in the cooler temperatures of the evening when the flowers open fully. Their scent is also particularly pervasive in the evening dampness and carries much further than many day scents. In nature, many of these species predominate in sheltered valleys where the scent is contained, along with the pollinators, giving a clue as to how best to site them in our gardens.

Since, in general, flowers also produce perfume as a strategy to attract instead of producing strong flower colour, it is not an easy task to produce a brightly coloured scented garden. Rely instead on paler colours. Many modern hybrids have been bred for strong colour and have lost fragrance in the process – an example is the popular tobacco plant now available in

PALE FLOWERS ARE USUALLY THE MOST SCENTED. CLIMBERS DELIVER PERFUME AT NOSE LEVEL.

dwarf strains of good colour, but for perfume you would need to obtain the species *Nicotiana alata* or *N. sylvestris*.

Not all flowers produce scent that is attractive to humans. Since they are trying to attract flies or other insects they may emit the scent of decay in imitation of the decaying food sources of those insects. Many members of the arum family and tree members of the rose family (such as hawthorn, pyracantha and the bird cherry) do this and should always be planted well away from the house and never used as cut flowers.

Not all scent in plants is produced in flowers. Many of the essential oils are contained in the leaves and stems and are given off when the tissue is bruised or crushed. Many of these species can be used to enhance sensory qualities in gardens with particular benefits to people with visual impairment. From the plant's point of view, these substances are there to act as defence against pest attack and to repel animals from browsing. Many species originate from arid

THE EVERGREEN HONEYSUCKLE, *LONICERA JAPONICA* 'HALLIANA', (OPPOSITE) HAS ONE OF THE STRONGEST PERFUMES IN THE GENUS.

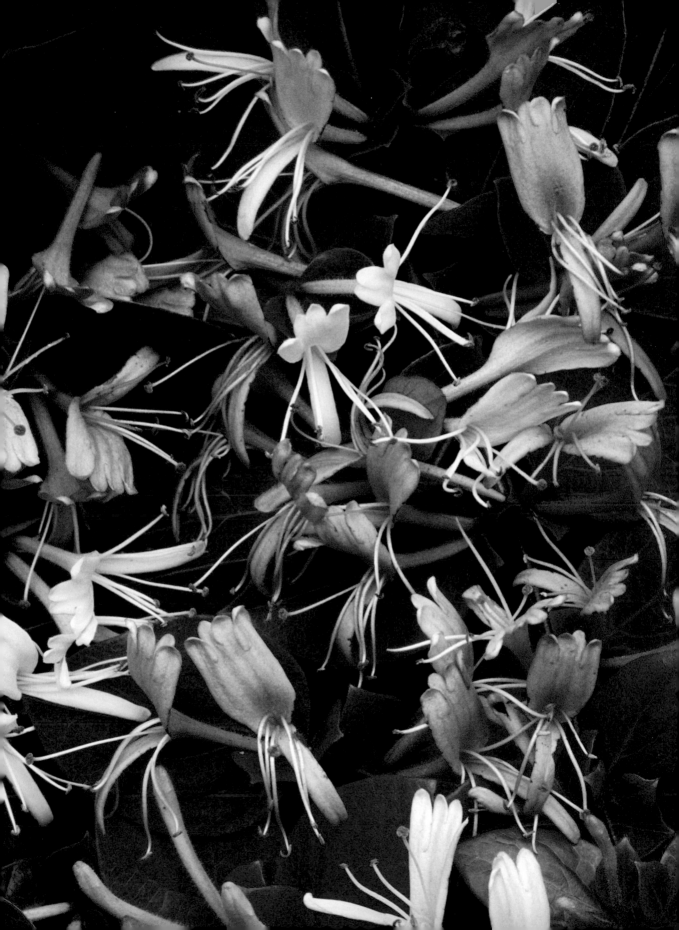

HIGHLY SCENTED PLANTS

Daphne odora 'Aureo Marginata'

One of the easiest daphnes to grow, this produces a delicious spicy-lemon scent from its early spring flowers. It is evergreen, will grow to 1.2 × 1.2m (4 × 4ft) and does best in a warm sheltered position in well-drained soil. The scent carries well. *Hardiness zone 7.*

Dianthus 'Mrs Sinkins'

This pink produces double white flowers with a strong clove scent in midsummer from a mat of evergreen, grey-green foliage. Stems rise to 30cm (1ft) and it will spread to 45cm (18in). Take cuttings in spring and replace the old plants every few years as they are naturally short-lived. A sunny position is essential and limey well-drained soil is preferred. *Hardiness zone 3.*

Heliotropium Heliotrope

Heliotrope is commonly known as cherry pie, which is a good description of its scent, though it is also likened to marzipan. The cultivars are tender perennial plants normally raised as annuals from seed sown under glass in spring and bedded out in pots or containers placed where the nose can best appreciate them. Heights range from 15 × 15cm (6 × 6in) to 45 × 30cm (18 × 12in). *Hardiness zone 10.*

Hyacinthus orientalis Hyacinth

Hyacinths are often bought as 'prepared' bulbs for planting in early autumn for early flowering indoors. They can also be bought, untreated, for massing in the flower garden for their scent, which peaks in mid to late spring. Growing them in a contained space such as a courtyard or hedged area will contain and thus concentrate their scent. Plant bulbs with the depth of the bulb above them, in well-drained soils in sun. Hyacinths will not naturalize as effectively as narcissi and need to be replaced every few years – or yearly. Height to 23cm (9in). *Hardiness zone 8.*

Lilium regale Regal lily

This is one of the finest species of lilies for scent (lily cultivars such as 'Casablanca' may have an even sweeter scent – but are less hardy). Regal lilies will grow to 1.2m × 23cm (4ft × 9in) from bulbs planted at twice their depth (to allow for rooting out from the stem above the bulb) in autumn or early spring. They will naturalize and even self-seed, where happy, in good soil in sun. *Hardiness zone 5.*

Nicotiana alata Tobacco

This is a half-hardy annual growing to 1m × 30cm (3ft × 1ft). Sow the seed in spring under glass, and plant out when all risk of frost is past. It does best in semi-shade, but try to choose areas where you can enjoy the fragrance on summer evenings when the flowers open. *Hardiness zone 7.*

Philadelphus

These deciduous shrubs produce lemon-scented white flowers, single or double, in midsummer. They vary in height from 60 × 60cm (2 × 2ft) in

ROSA PRIMULA (OPPOSITE) HAS LEAVES THAT RELEASE FRAGRANCE AFTER RAIN.

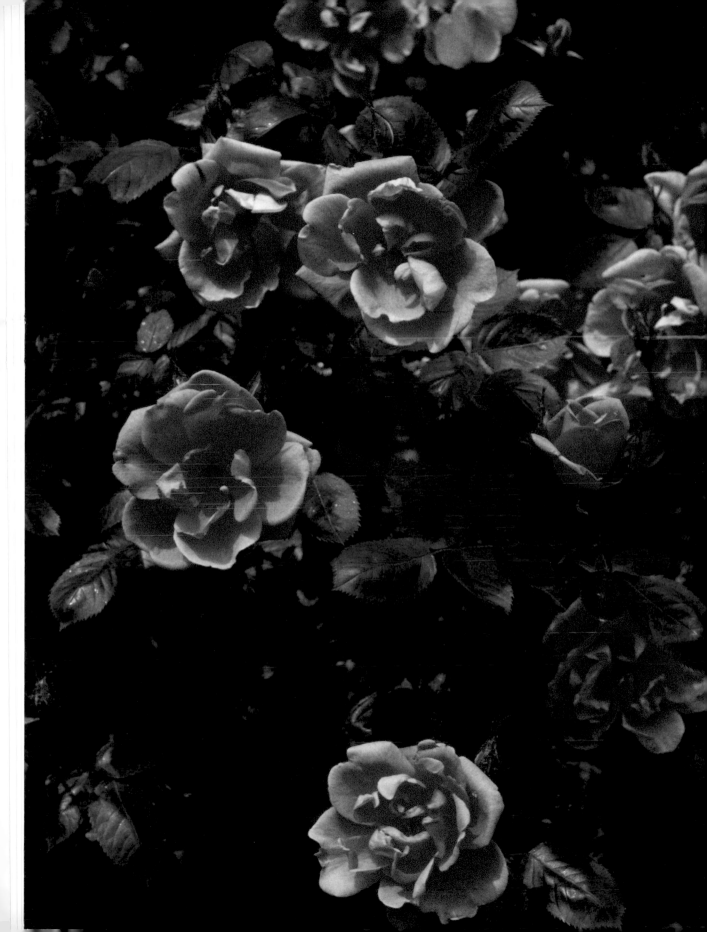

PLANTS TO ENJOY TOUCHING

Acer capillipes Snake bark maple

The common name of this maple comes from its fine, striated bark. The tree grows to 7.5 × 6m (25 × 20ft) in deep, fertile soil in a sheltered position; like most maples, the colour of the autumn foliage is spectacular. *Hardiness zone 5.*

Acer griseum Paper bark maple

The flaking, peeling bark of this maple is curious to touch; and, as an added bonus, the bark is a rich brown colour, especially fine when backlit against the sun, when it matches the orange glow of the autumn foliage. The tree is slow growing to 5 × 3m (16 × 10ft). *Hardiness zone 5.*

Achillea filipendulina 'Gold Plate'

This herbaceous perennial will grow to 1–2 × 1m (3–4 × 3ft) and produces very flat flowers of a texture that is interesting to the palm of the hand. It needs full sun but tolerates any well-drained soil. *Hardiness zone 3.*

Allium giganteum Giant ornamental onion

This will grow to 1–1.5m × 30cm (3–5 × 1ft) from bulbs planted in autumn or spring. It produces rich purple, dense, globular flower heads. Try cupping them in your hand. Full sun is required. *Hardiness zone 8.*

Antirrhinum majus 'Nanum Compactum' Snapdragon

Antirrhinums are plants which many children will have played with, squeezing the side of each flower to make them gape. They have a velvety texture. This cultivar grows to 23 × 23cm (9 × 9in). Grow as half-hardy annuals, raising seedlings under glass from seed sown in spring. Plant out in early summer when all risk of frost is past. *Hardiness zone 7.*

Buddleja crispa

This is a buddleja with velvety, white-felted leaves and stems which are inviting to touch. It will grow to 3 × 2.5m (10 × 8ft) but needs a protected, sunny position. *Hardiness zone 8.*

Centaurea dealbata Perennial cornflower

This perennial, which grows to 60 × 60cm (2 × 2ft), produces blue flowers that are followed by papery seed-heads. It is extremely easy to grow in sun in any soil. *Hardiness zone 3.*

Cosmos bipinnatus cultivars

These annuals grow to 1.2m × 45cm (4ft × 18in) and produce flowers with satin-sheened petals (in a variety of colours from white to pink and purple). Seed should be direct sown in late spring in poor soil in sun for a summer display. *Hardiness zone 8.*

Crambe maritime Seakale

This perennial, used as a vegetable, produces waxy, glaucous leaves which help it survive in a maritime habitat. It grows to 60 × 90cm (2 × 3ft). *Hardiness zone 5.*

CENTAUREA DEALBATA HAS SEED-HEADS WITH AN INTERESTING PAPERY TEXTURE.

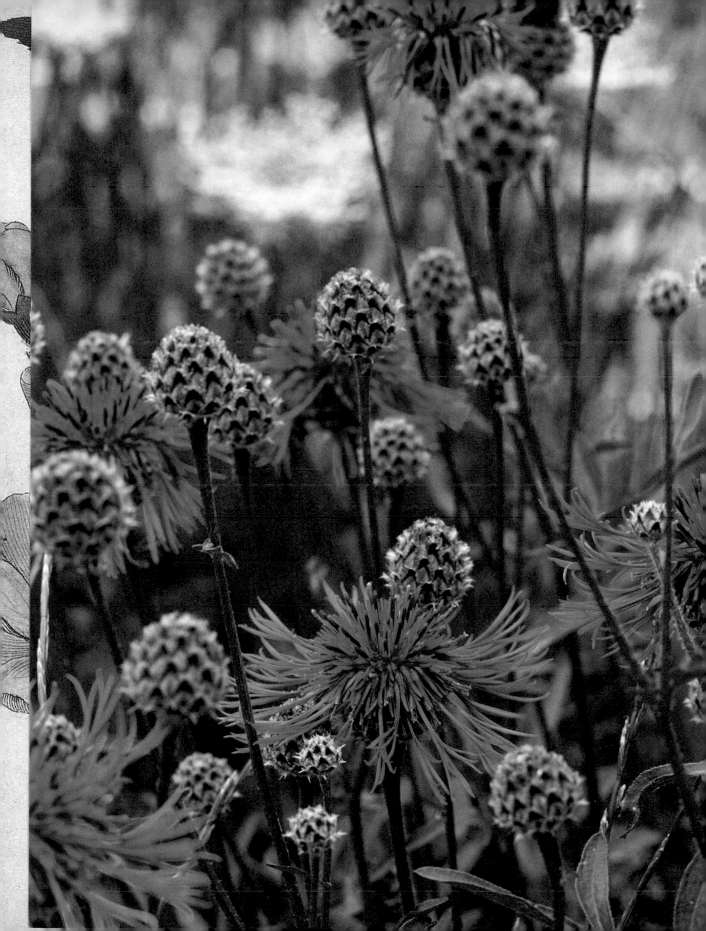

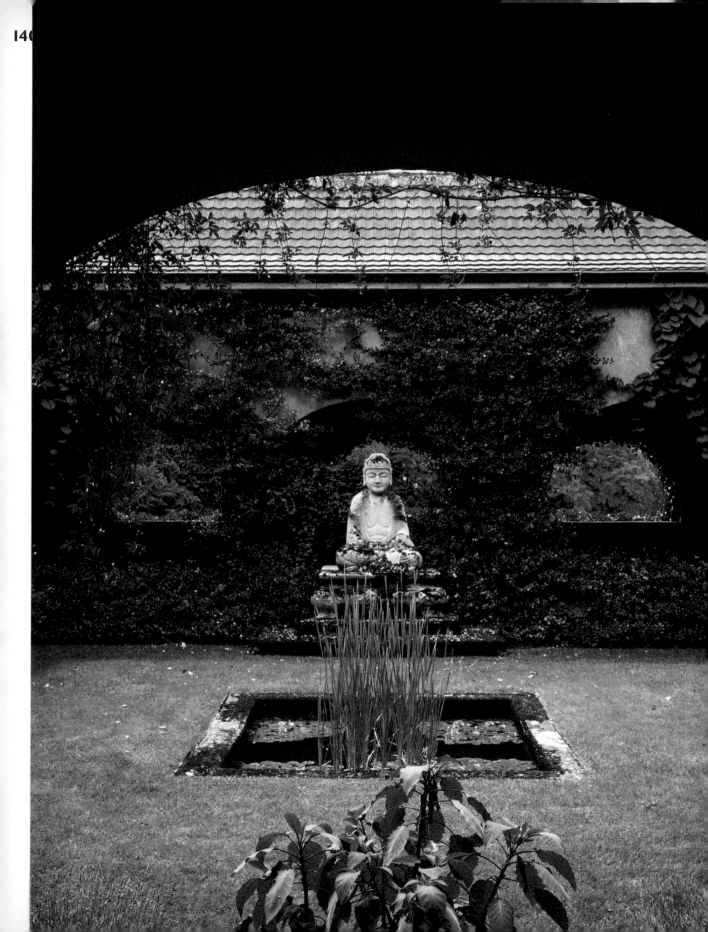

A SPIRITUAL
HAVEN

THROUGHOUT HISTORY THE GARDEN HAS HELD A CENTRAL PLACE IN THE SPIRITUAL QUEST FOR PARADISE AND THE CONCEPT OF A GARDEN AS A SANCTUARY APPEARS IN MOST OF THE WORLD'S great religions. Our own gardens are sanctuaries in a similar way, sources of refreshment, growth, change and peace. That they can be places of healing is proven in that it has been shown quite conclusively that hospital patients recover more quickly when they have a view of a garden.

For many people, a garden is a place of absorbing interest totally different from their workaday lives, a place that allows them to develop aspects of their personalities that may be denied elsewhere.

A CALM, ENCLOSED GARDEN HAS A SPIRITUAL QUALITY WITH OR WITHOUT ANY OBVIOUS RELIGIOUS REFERENCE.

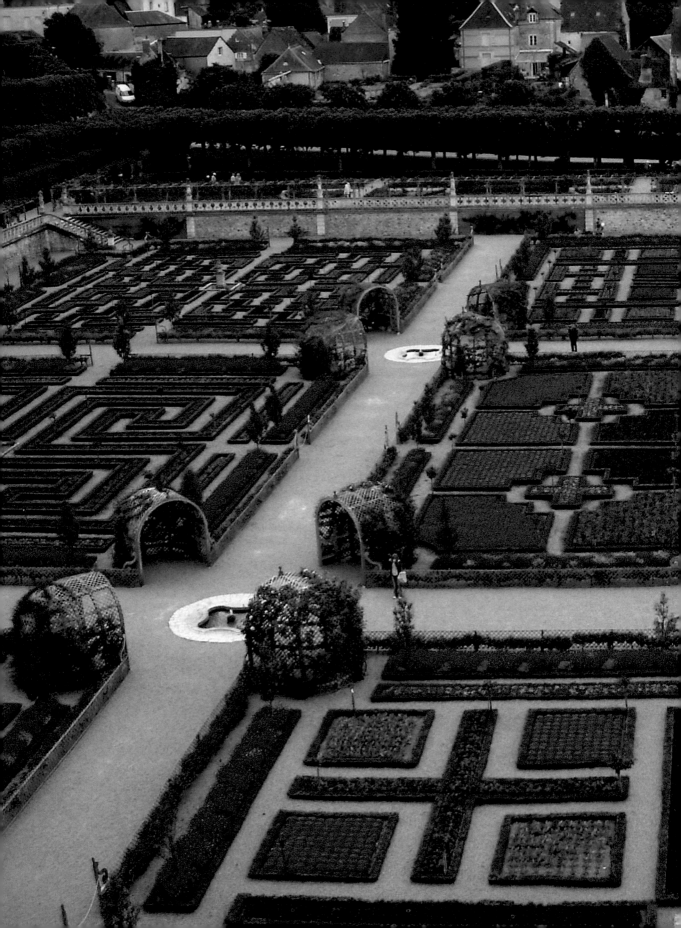

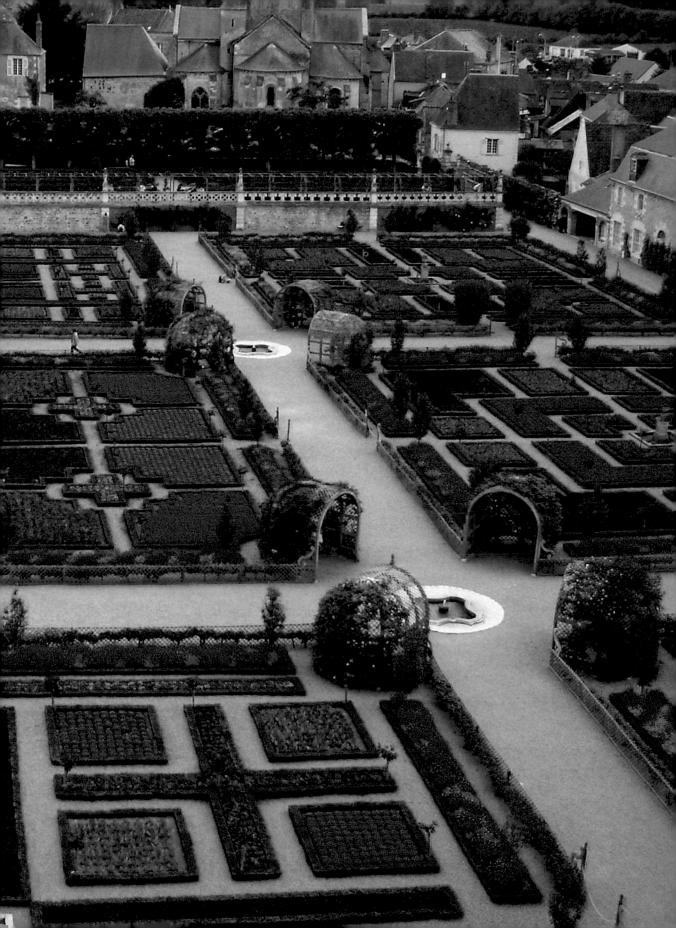

DISCOVERING YOUR OWN STYLE

The way that you design your garden can play an important role in your view of the natural world and how you wish to interact with it, and can also affirm your personality in a healing sense, giving you a chance to create a living space just as you wish it to be. Looking at the history of garden design and visiting other gardens are two of the best ways to help you to form ideas for the sort of garden you would like yourself and the particular ambience and effect you wish to create there.

Great traditions of garden design have tended both to reflect a national identity and to show people's individual view of their relation to nature. Attitudes and tastes have tended to veer between attempts to control nature and letting it hold sway. The great seventeenth-century French and Dutch gardens, such as those at the palaces of Versailles, near Paris, and Het Loo, in Apeldoorn, Holland, with their intricate formal parterres, long allées, clipped evergreens and perfect symmetry, express total control over nature, almost a desire to keep it at bay. In France many formal gardens expressed royal power and were made by armies often under the direction of the great garden creator André Le Nôtre.

The eighteenth-century movement that swept away all traces of formality in English gardens was partly a liberal reaction to autocratic French rigidity, and partly a nostalgic attempt to recreate the classical landscapes of Greece and

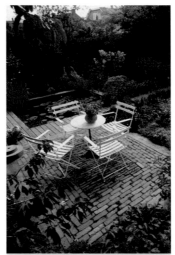

DOMESTIC GARDENS ARE PERSONAL LIVING SPACES. HERE PLANTS ARE A BACKDROP TO CONVIVIALITY.

Rome in which visitors could be free to form their own impressions. The essential concern was not to impose order and regularity on a site, but to let the nature of the site express itself. The influential poet Alexander Pope maintained that 'All gardening is landscape painting', and designers such as William Kent, Lancelot 'Capability' Brown and Charles Bridgeman remodelled the English landscape much as if they were artists.

Great landscape gardens such as Stowe, in Buckinghamshire, and Rousham, in Oxfordshire, influenced some of the formal gardens of Tuscany, where much of the formality was replaced by lawns, as at the Villa Torrigiani, Lucca, as well as gardens in France and Germany. In the USA the English landscape movement inspired Thomas Jefferson, whose garden at Monticello, Virginia, started in 1769, has now been restored.

By the beginning of the nineteenth century another reappraisal of attitudes to nature,

A GARDEN TO POTTER IN (OPPOSITE). FREEDOM TO INDULGE UNASSIGNED
TIME IS A VITAL ATTRIBUTE OF MANY GARDENS TODAY.

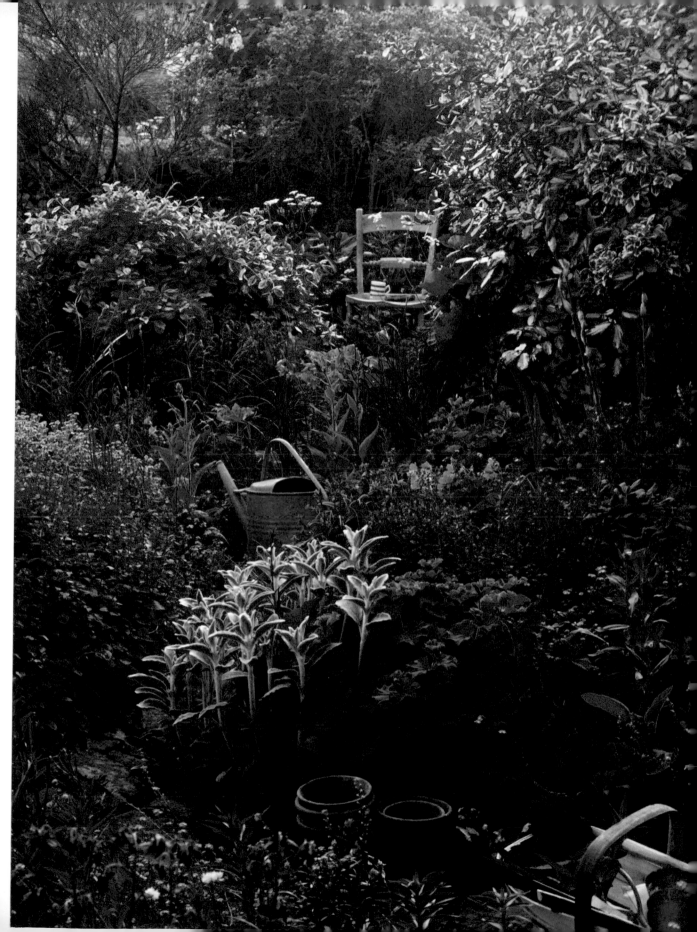

DESIGNING A SMALL GARDEN

When you begin to design a garden, you have first to think about your ideas and ideals, and then balance these with the constraints of the site, the size of your budget and how much time you want to give to gardening. In general, gardens with structure, i.e. those with a good deal of hard surfaces, are usually easier and less time consuming to maintain than those with a mass of plants. This would satisfy those short of time but it would frustrate the keen plantsman or woman.

As well as the basic style you want to create, you should think about how you want to use the garden, and then list any particular features that you know you want to include, such as a pergola, a pond, a seating area, a sundial or containers. Take time – and visit as many gardens as you can – to gather your thoughts, and take time to get to know the site: you should consider its aspect (the amount of shade and where it falls), its type of soil, and other considerations such as noisy neighbours that you might want to block out with high fences or hedges.

Advice on designing specific types of garden and garden features, such as wildlife gardens and water features, are dealt with on pages 162 and 120 respectively. Easy ways to give immediate distinctive character to a garden are discussed on pages 172–4. Specific ideas on the use of colour, scent, sound and texture are given on pages 102, 122, 116 and 134.

Once you have decided on the basic

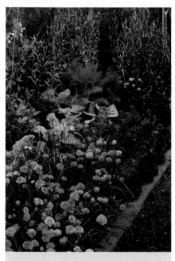

KEEN GARDENERS WILL WANT ANY AVAILABLE SPACE TO BE STUFFED WITH PLANTS.

approach, you will need to measure your site and transfer your measurements to a paper sketch plan from which your final design can be accurately drawn. The best way to do this is with a 30-metre landscape architect's tape. Measure a base line, that is the longest unbroken line that can be marked out on the site, and mark all your measurements against this. Existing trees and other features that you wish to retain can be accurately plotted by measuring from two points and describing intersecting arcs with a pair of compasses to mark the position exactly.

You may need to make minor adjustments to levels within the site. Insert a peg into the ground a short distance away from the level you have chosen to match, such as a doorstep. Using a wooden lath to rest on the peg and doorstep, check with a spirit level that the peg is level. Continue to measure around the site with further pegs. By measuring from these permanent levels to the existing soil level you can work out how much soil, hardcore, etc. you will

A PERFECTLY DESIGNED SHOWPIECE (OPPOSITE). VISITING GARDENS OR GARDEN SHOWS IS A GOOD WAY TO GARNER IDEAS.

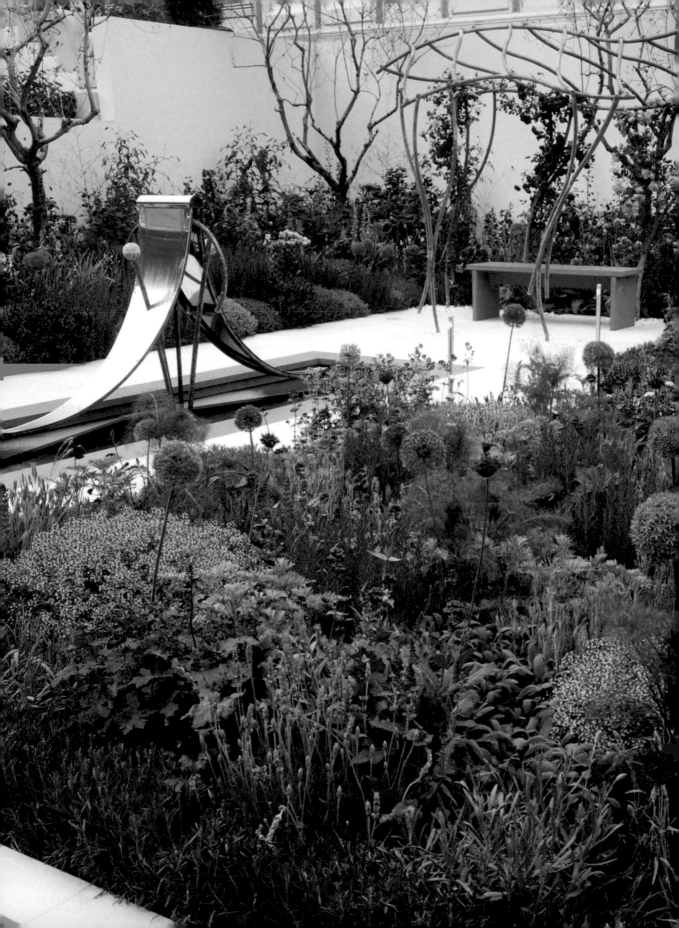

need to achieve a final true level. Transfer all this information to a plan drawn at 1:50 or 1:100 scale depending on the size of the garden, with a cross-section plan to show the levels.

Now experiment on a sketch plan to produce a design that is pleasing to your eye and has the right mix of 'hardworks', such as paths and paving, and planting areas. Think about the pattern the beds will form, especially if the garden can be viewed from above, and how one enters and moves around the garden. If you wish to incorporate seating, arbours, terracotta pots, statuary or other features that will affect the ground plan, decide whether they are to be placed symmetrically or singly as focal points within the garden. Remember to leave enough room to move into or around these features freely so that they do not cause obstruction.

Paths and paving

The paths and paving in a garden form its basic ground plan, although it is possible, especially in a formal garden, to emphasize the layout with formally clipped plants. Reclaimed York stone, or one of the better textured modern substitutes, is an excellent but expensive choice for paving, which should be laid on a 7.5cm (3in) deep bed of hardcore blinded over with sand to form a level and secure base.

Brick is a good alternative, especially in a very small garden, and can be laid in a variety of patterns – basket-weave or herringbone, for example – that can look very attractive. If you go for this option, you must use weatherproof bricks specially made for exterior use. More interest at ground level can be created by mixing materials; for example, stone can be varied with sections of

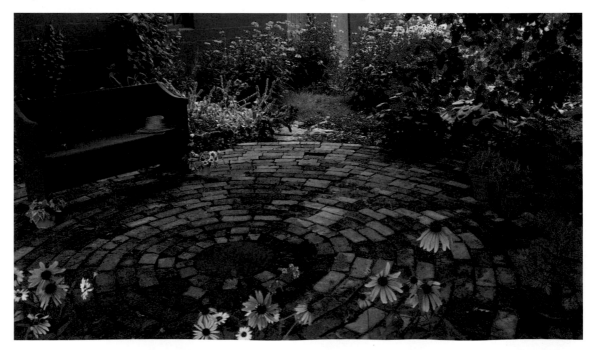

USING WEATHERPROOF BRICK FOR A SEATING AREA. DESIGNING CIRCLES WITHIN SQUARE OR RECTANGULAR PLOTS WILL INCREASE THE PERCEPTION OF THEIR WIDTH.

cobbles or areas of brick. But do not use too many variants or the effect may become unsettling.

For a cheaper option you can use pea gravel. Lay a 7.5cm (3in) hardcore base, top this off with coarse gravel and then lay 2.5–4cm (1–1½ in) of dry 'hoggin' (a mix of stone and clay which will set hard). Roll it with a heavy roller and then spread your gravel onto this. It is worth the time and trouble at this stage as a well-laid gravel path will last for a good many years. Alternatively, lay a geotextile membrane on top of your hardcore base and simply top with pea gravel.

For some years now, wooden decking has become a fashionable alternative to paving and is easily obtainable in self-assembly kits. It is particularly appropriate around timber-framed or timber-clad buildings – indeed, this was its original use. Make sure the timber is from a sustainable source.

Enclosure and division

The choice of the means to enclose or divide up your garden will depend upon your taste, but also upon your budget. Walls, fencing and hedges all have advantages and disadvantages. Walls are permanent but very costly; fencing is cheaper, versatile, and quicker to install, but has a designated life before it needs replacing (although its life can be extended by attaching it to posts that are cemented in to the ground or, more permanently, to posts bolted onto metal stakes that do not rot). Hedges are cheap to put in and can make some of the best backgrounds for planting, but take time to establish and require yearly maintenance.

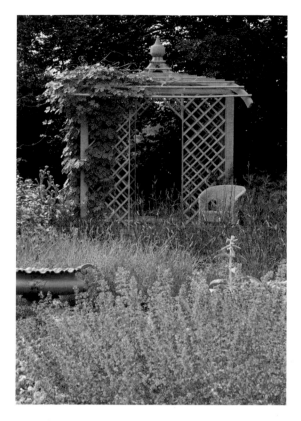

If you have restricted space and want to create a formal atmosphere and vertical accent, consider using trellis edging, or even low ironwork edging round your beds. These take up little ground horizontally but create a feeling of formal enclosure. Divisions can be combined with the means to provide places for shade, rest and relaxation, in pergolas and arbours.

Walls, fences, pergolas and arbours can all be clothed in plants. If your design is formal make sure that your selection of plants does not overwhelm the design by its lushness. Part of the pleasure of formal gardens is their structure, so make sure that the planting complements rather than obscures it.

ARBOURS ARE USEFUL FEATURES IN GARDENS, PROVIDING SHADE, VERTICALITY IN THE LANDSCAPE AND AN OPPORTUNITY TO GROW CLIMBING PLANTS.

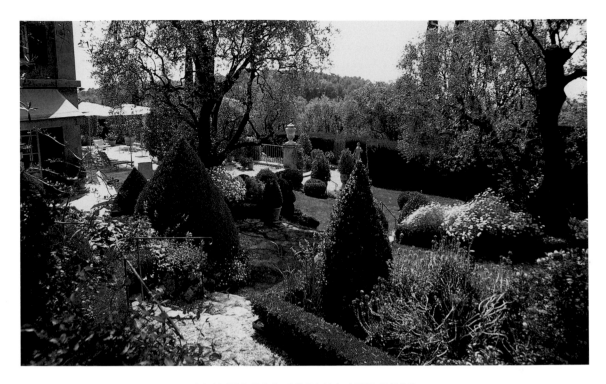

PLANTS FOR FORMAL HEDGING

Buxus sempervirens Box

This is an evergreen, slow-growing British native suitable for chalky soil. It usually needs clipping twice annually, once in early summer, and again in early autumn. The dwarf form *B. s.* 'Suffruticosa' is suitable for low hedges in parterres and to edge and retain soil in other formal beds. *Hardiness zone 5.*

Carpinus betulus Hornbeam

Hornbeam is often planted 'where beech won't do', i.e. in moister soils than beech would tolerate. Like beech, it will often retain its shrivelled, caramel-coloured leaves in winter. Trim annually in late summer. *Hardiness zone 5.*

Elaeagnus

These salt-tolerant shrubs are excellent for hedging in coastal areas and bear fragrant flowers (scented of lily-of-the-valley). The hybrid *E. × ebbingei* is evergreen. *E. commutata* is deciduous but very useful on poor, sandy soils, though it can be invasive. *Both hardy to zone 2.*

Fagus sylvatica Beech

A deciduous British native, this is especially suitable for light chalky soils. It has the attractive habit of retaining its juvenile leaves (though browned) throughout winter. Clip yearly in late summer. *Hardiness zone 5.*

BOX IS THE MOST COMMON EVERGREEN FOR EDGING FORMAL BEDS AND
YEW FOR CREATING FORMAL HEDGES AND TOPIARY.

Ilex Holly

Hollies are evergreen and will make dense hedges but are slow-growing so you need to be patient. It is always best to plant young, container-grown plants as hollies resent root disturbance. *I. × alta-clarensis* is a hybrid which tolerates polluted perimeters (for example against roads) and can be used at the seaside too. There are many cultivars to choose from, some variegated, some less spiny than others. Only female forms will berry (the large berries of *I. aquifolium* are particularly attractive to birds). *Hardy to zone 6.*

Ligustrum ovalifolium Privet

The staple, more-or-less evergreen hedging plant requires clipping at least three times a year and has little to recommend it unless you want a golden hedge, in which case grow the clones 'Aureum' or 'Lemon and Lime'. *Hardiness zone 5.*

Quercus ilex Holm oak

This evergreen species will make a dense hedge in warm regions, requiring clipping in late summer. *Hardy to zone 7.*

Taxus baccata Yew

Yew is the classic evergreen hedging plant for formal gardens and also for topiary (or where topiary is included in a hedge). Yew is faster growing than most people think and is an excellent choice for limey soils. It will also rejuvenate very successfully if cut back hard in late summer. Annual trimming is required in late summer – the cuttings may be saleable to pharmaceutical companies manufacturing the anti-cancer taxol drugs. Remember, yew foliage and seed is poisonous if eaten by humans or livestock (although the fleshy arils surrounding the seeds are not poisonous and are often stripped by birds). *Hardiness zone 6.*

Thuja plicata Western red cedar

This conifer is evergreen with foliage scented attractively of pineapple. It is a far better, more controllable, hedging plant than the ubiquitous Leyland cypress. It does best in moist areas. Clip in late summer. *Hardiness zone 6.*

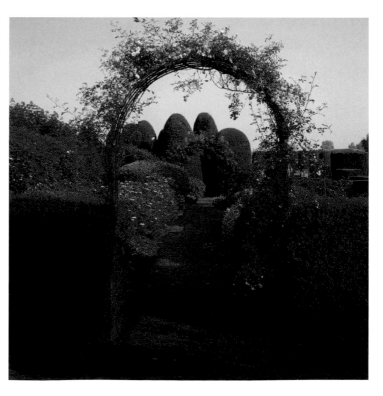

AN INFORMAL ROSE ARCH AMID A BOX HEDGE FRAMES
FORMALLY CLIPPED YEWS IN THE DISTANCE.

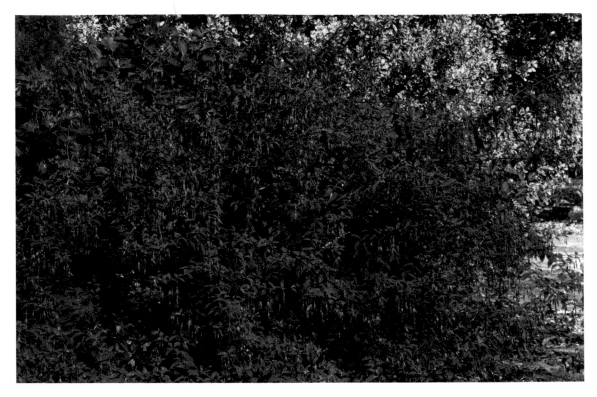

PLANTS FOR INFORMAL HEDGING

Amelanchier lamarckii
This is often grown as a free-standing deciduous shrub but makes a good informal hedge with the double advantage of white flowers in spring emerging from coppery young foliage, followed by excellent autumn colour. *Hardiness zone 4.*

Berberis Barberry
The barberries make excellent, dense, thorny hedges. Most of them have yellow or orange flowers and berry freely. Good evergreen species include *B. gagnepainii*, *B. darwinii* and the hybrid *B.* × *stenophylla* (which also provides good berries for birds). The deciduous *B. thunbergii* has some attractive purple-leaved forms and also a dwarf form for low hedges, *B. thunbergii* 'Atropurpurea Nana'. Trim all these in late summer. *Hardiness zones 5, 7, 5 and 4 respectively.*

Chaenomeles Flowering quince, or Japonica
These deciduous shrubs make useful thorny hedges with spring flowers in colours from red to salmon-pink. Most cultivars are derived from *C. speciosa. Hardiness zone 5.*

Cotoneaster lacteus and *Cotoneaster salicifolius*
Both these evergreen shrubs are useful, mostly

FUCHSIA MAGELLANICA MAKES A FLORIFEROUS HEDGE FOR MILD AREAS
AND FLOWERS FROM JULY ONWARDS.

for forming large hedges for the use of wildlife because of their berries. Prune to shape in late winter. *Hardiness zone 6.*

Crataegus monogyna Hawthorn

A thorny hedging plant useful for its early white flowers and autumn colour. The berries attract birds. *Hardiness zone 5.*

Escallonia

These are useful evergreen shrubs for hedges in maritime areas. *E. rubra* var. *macrantha* produces red flowers. Prune to shape after flowering. *Hardiness zone 8.*

Fuchsia

F. magellanica and its forms and cultivars make excellent, floriferous deciduous hedges in warm regions. Plant them where they will get good moisture. *Hardiness zone 6.*

Hydrangea macrophylla and Hydrangea serrata

Both the 'mophead' and the 'lacecap' flowering types of hydrangea make informal hedges, providing useful late-summer colour. Do not remove the dead flower heads until early spring. All hydrangeas need moist soil, and do best in partial shade. *Hardy to zones 5 and 6 respectively.*

Olearia Daisy bush

These Australasian evergreens make good hedges, and are especially suitable for maritime gardens. Suitable species include *O. macrodonta* and the hybrid *O.* × *haastii*, both with white flowers; *hardy to zone 8.*

Potentilla fruticosa

These are useful plants for low, informal hedges to 6ocm (2ft), although they are deciduous. They are available in flower colours ranging from white through to yellow to pink and red. They prefer sun and poor soil. Trim in spring. *Hardiness zone 5.*

Pyracantha Firethorn

These are useful for impenetrable hedging and have the triple benefit of being evergreen, spring flowering and having berries in the autumn that are of value to birds. Many cultivars are available in different berry colours. Ask for forms that are resistant to fireblight. *Hardiness zones 7 or 8.*

Rosa rugosa Rose

This rose makes an excellent deciduous hedge, erect and prickly with forms in white, red or pink followed by colourful hips. *Extremely hardy – to zone 2.*

PYRACANTHAS ARE GOOD BOTH FOR BURGLAR-DETERRING HEDGES AND FOR WILDLIFE.

MAKING A WILDLIFE GARDEN

Having contact with other living creatures is often considered healing (although studies on this have usually been done in the context of pets). It is a strange paradox that whereas people used to go into the countryside to seek contact with and observe wildlife, modern farming practices have forced wildlife itself into cities. The urban garden can become a refuge for all sorts of birds, mammals and invertebrates and this contact with nature can be enjoyed at first hand by anyone with a small patch of land and some basic hints on how to encourage living creatures. The 'design' of gardens for this purpose is therefore really 'designing for habitat'.

If you consider the area covered by domestic gardens, good practices here could form the basis of a huge 'nature reserve' where wildlife has a sanctuary against pesticide use and habitat loss. There are many ways you can encourage creatures to visit (for example, by providing food and nest boxes for birds) but it is much more exciting to try to recreate a small area of a natural habitat. This means understanding something of ecology and the various food chains necessary to make the habitat fully functional.

There are a number of elements necessary to a wildlife garden for it to be ecologically successful: a nectar border to attract butterflies and moths; a pond for native species of fish and invertebrates, with an area for moisture-loving plants next to it; a meadow or flowery bank (preferably edged with a hedge); and an area representative of the edge of a wood-

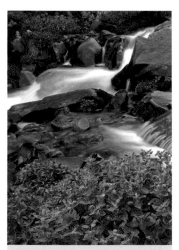

WATER IN A GARDEN WILL ALWAYS ATTRACT WILDLIFE AND ALSO ALLOWS THE PLANTING OF MARGINAL AND MOISTURE-LOVING PLANTS.

land, a very diverse and species-rich environment.

The nectar border is the element closest to familiar garden design and you should site this in a sunny, sheltered position preferably close to, and easily viewed from, the house. Select plants from the species listed on page 164.

A pond can be created using a liner (see page 170), and you can extend the liner (punctured in a few places) under an adjacent bed to create an area with impeded drainage. This makes an excellent wetland habitat that you can plant with species such as the marsh marigold (*Caltha palustris*), meadowsweet (*Filipendula ulmaria*), monkey flower (*Mimulus guttatus*), purple loosestrife (*Lythrum salicaria*) and yellow flag (*Iris pseudacorus*), all of which are very colourful as well as attractive to insects.

Many people like the idea of wildflower gardening and if you are prepared to forgo a lawn,

CORNFIELD 'WEEDS' (USUALLY NOW SUPPRESSED BY HERBICIDES IN CROPPED FIELDS) PROVIDE A POPULAR DISPLAY AT THE EDEN PROJECT (OPPOSITE).

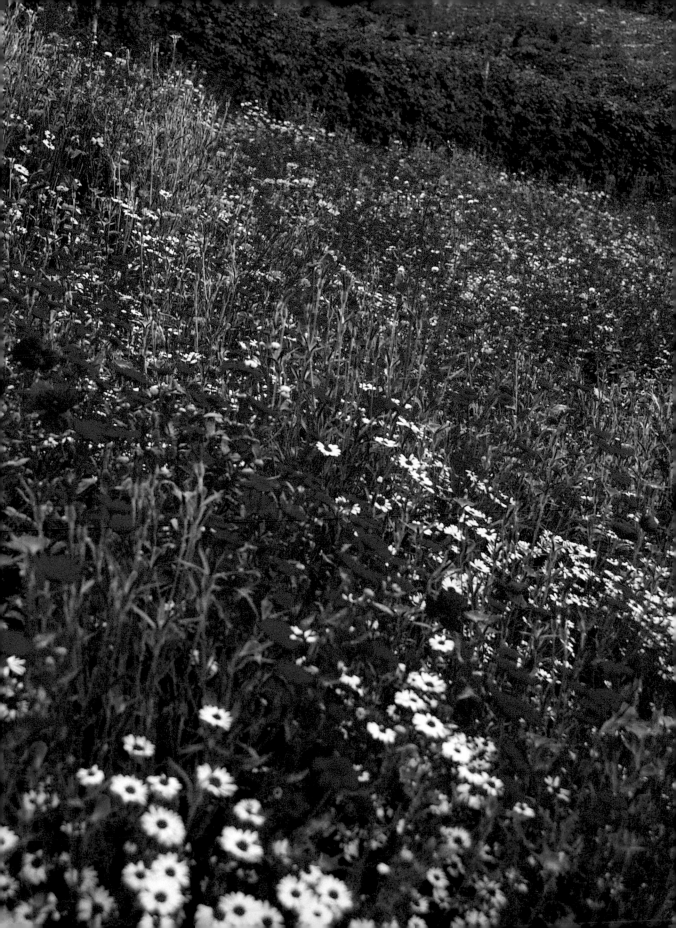

and providing your soil is of fairly low fertility, you could consider sowing a wildflower meadow. There are various seed mixtures specially prepared for this. The wildflower mixtures at the Eden Project have been hugely successful, both in the biomes and outside. A meadow would normally need to be mown once in late summer, but you can provide access by regularly mowing an informal path through it weekly.

Hedgerow habitats have been decimated by the drive for agricultural efficiency. You can imitate a hedgerow environment by planting a mixed hedge of native species, rather than the ubiquitous privet or Leyland cypress. In Britain plant species such as blackthorn (*Prunus spinosa*), sea buckthorn (*Hippophae rhamnoides*), dogwood (*Cornus sanguinea*), elder (*Sambucus nigra*), hawthorn (*Crataegus monogyna*), hazel (*Corylus avellana*) and dog rose (*Rosa canina*) make good hedges and provide berries and fruits for wildlife. Trim the hedge in late winter when in least use by birds and mammals.

If you have a large enough space, you might like to create an area to imitate a woodland edge. Use native trees and shrubs to provide shade, and import logs and stumps or make a woodpile that can rot and provide habitats for insects and invertebrates. Once an area is established you can underplant it with nursery-produced bluebells (*Hyacinthoides non-scripta*), wood anemones (*Anemone nemorosa*), herb paris (*Paris quadrifolia*) and other native flowers of the forest floor. Use

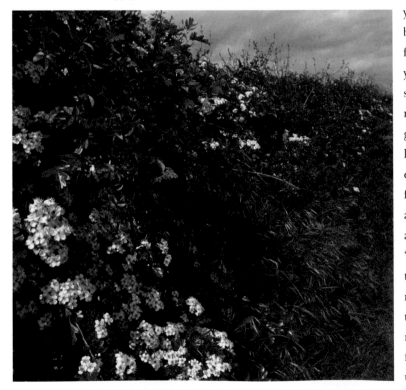

your woodland area to site nest boxes and you will probably find that birds will use them if you have encouraged the provision of food for them by your management of the rest of the garden. You can also encourage hedgehogs (wonderful destroyers of slugs) by leaving a box filled with straw in a wooded area of the garden. Hedgehogs are territorial and if one 'adopts' you, nothing is nicer than feeding it pet food at night and feeling honoured by the visits. This contact with nature can be a real refuge from the artificiality of much urban living.

HEDGEROWS PROVIDE VITAL FOOD AND REFUGE FOR BIRDS AND MAMMALS. USE NATIVE PLANTS WHERE POSSIBLE.

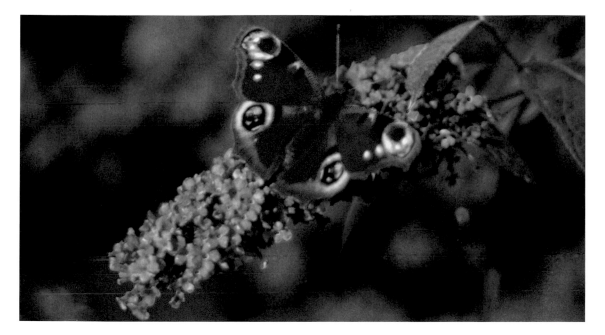

PLANTS TO ENCOURAGE BUTTERFLIES AND OTHER INSECTS

Agrostemma githago Corncockle

This is a British native cornfield annual growing to 60cm (2ft) which is now endangered due to farming practices. Sow in open ground in spring and collect seed to sow again annually. *Hardiness zone 7.*

Buddleja davidii Butterfly bush

This deciduous shrub, which grows to 2 × 2m (6 × 6ft), requires hard pruning (coppicing) in mid spring to encourage flowering on current year's growth in late summer. It is not fussy about soil but prefers good drainage. *Hardiness zone 5.*

Caryopteris x *clandonensis*

This small deciduous shrub, reaching 1 × 1m (3 × 3ft), has neat grey foliage and quantities of lavender-blue flowers in late summer. It needs full sun and to be pruned in the same way as buddlejas. *Hardiness zone 7.*

Ceanothus Californian lilac

Most of these shrubs are prized for their clouds of blue flowers, which are particularly attractive to bees. They grow to 2–4 × 2m (6–12 × 6ft) and need full sun and good drainage. No pruning is usually required. *Hardiness zones 7–8, depending on variety.*

Centaurea cyanus Cornflower

A British native annual, it produces its fine blue flowers on stems to 45cm (18in). Treat in the same way as *Agrostemma githago. Hardiness zone 7.*

A TORTOISESHELL BUTTERFLY ON A *BUDDLEJA DAVIDII* CULTIVAR,
AN EXCELLENT NECTAR SHRUB.

MAKING POOLS FOR CONTEMPLATION

Pools of water exert an irresistible fascination. We respond to water as a life-giver and as a focal point for tranquil contemplation. Nowhere is this truer than in China, where still water in a garden is used to express serenity. A flat sheet of water is also used there as a complement to the vertical elements of the garden in the Chinese quest for balance in all things.

Throughout the centuries and all over the world, garden designers have used still water for its power to reflect. In eighteenth-century Britain, 'Capability' Brown designed huge 'natural' lakes, which were in fact carefully contrived, in many of his great commissions, for example at Blenheim Palace, near Oxford. In the same era, the garden at Stourhead, Wiltshire, was designed by Henry Hoare around a large lake, to produce delightful reflections of classical temples. Today, it is also valued for the equally lovely reflections of autumn colour from the mature trees. In the USA a fine eighteenth-century water garden was created at Middleton Place, near Charleston, South Carolina, on the side of the Ashley River. Now restored to its former glory, it features many terraced lakes, probably inspired by the rice fields that made its owner, Henry Middleton, wealthy. At Dumbarton Oaks, near Washington, DC, there is a lovely formal pebble garden designed to be covered by a shallow sheet of water to enrich the colour of the stones and to

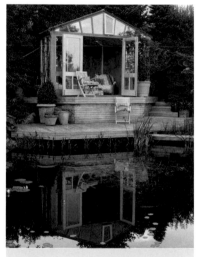

REFLECTIONS ARE ONE OF THE MAIN BENEFITS OF STILL WATER IN A GARDEN, WHETHER ON A GRAND OR DOMESTIC SCALE.

reflect the surrounding trees. Perhaps one of the most famous examples of still water is the lake created by the French Impressionist painter Claude Monet in the late nineteenth century in his garden at Giverny in northern France, to cultivate the water lilies that he adored to paint. Some water features have been constructed purely to mirror the outlines of particular buildings, such as the Taj Mahal at Agra in India.

If you want to make a reflective pool in your own garden, remember that pools can be high-maintenance features, requiring leaf fall to be cleared and fish protected from freezing conditions (and herons). If you do decide to go ahead, the first thing to consider is placing the pool. It is best sited where reflections can be easily visible from the various viewpoints in the garden, yet not where it will create unwanted reflections. It should be away from overhanging trees that will drop their leaves and pollute it, and if you want to stock it with aquatic plants, remember that they need good light to grow well.

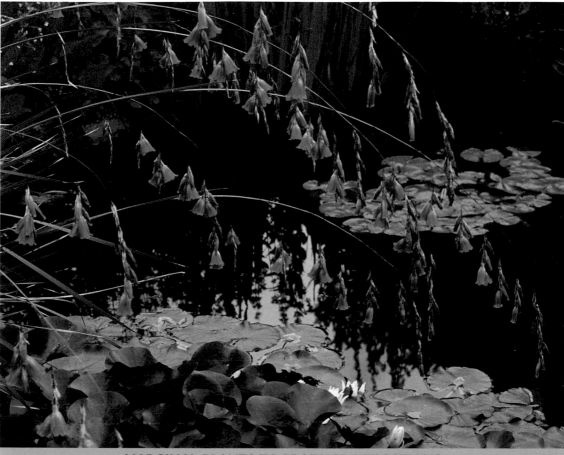

MARGINAL PLANTS TO PRODUCE REFLECTIONS

Aquatic plants can be very invasive, so you need to choose tall varieties that will cast reflections from the margins of a pool, rather than invade it. Here are some suggestions.

Common name	Botanical name	Height	Comment
Angel's Fishing Rod	*Dierama pulcherrimum*	1.2m (4ft)	Pretty, arching habit. Plant on bank.
Corkscrew Rush	*Juncus effusus* 'Spiralis'	45cm (1.5ft)	Curious twisted stems.
Dwarf Reedmace	*Typha minima*	30–75cm (1–2½ft)	Good for small pools.
Water Canna	*Thalia dealbata*	1.8m (6ft)	Needs winter protection.
Water Flag	*Iris pseudacorus*	1.5m (5ft)	Very erect habit, yellow flowers.
Water Iris	*Iris laevigata* varieties	75cm (2½ft)	Use where the Water Flag is too tall.
Zebra Sedge	*Scirpus tabernaemontani* 'Zebrinus'	1m (3ft)	Foliage banded green and white.

THE WELL-NAMED ANGEL'S FISHING ROD PRODUCES A SPECTACULAR DISPLAY IN JUNE.
IT HAILS FROM THE DRAKENSBURG MOUNTAINS IN SOUTH AFRICA.

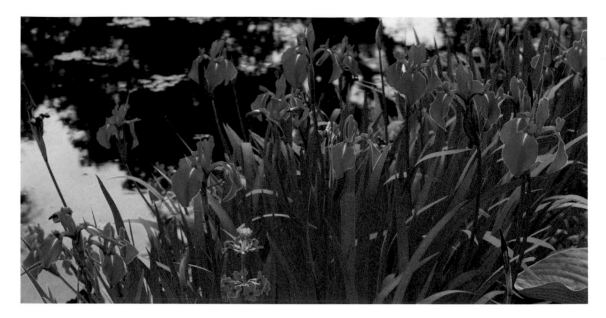

The surface area of the pool should be as generous as you can afford, and its shape should complement the design of your garden: a geometrical shape, positioned so that it is an integral part of the overall layout, suits a formal garden, whereas a pond with curved outlines works in an informal or wild garden. Do not obscure the edges of a formal pool with too many spreading plants – consider using erect iris or rushes – whereas more rampant plants around an informal pool will allow it to blend better into its surroundings.

There are three main methods of creating a pool: with a butyl rubber liner, a pre-formed (usually fibreglass) liner, and concrete. The easiest method is to use a good-quality liner, especially a black liner, which makes the water appear darker and more reflective. This is ideally suited to an informal design, but you can also use one to line a formal raised pool created from brickwork or concrete formwork. This type of raised pool may be more suitable to a small town garden or where toddlers need to be protected from falling in. (Any water is dangerous if there are young children about – pebble fountains are safest in family households. See pages 120–1.)

Water lilies need to be grown in still water. They are best planted in tubs of unsterilized loam weighted down with gravel and then sited in the water. Choose varieties that are suited in vigour to the size of the pool and the depth of the water (see page 171). Like most aquatic plants, they grow extremely quickly, and you may need to cull growth regularly to maintain the reflective area. Remember also that pools can become dangerous when completely covered with vegetation because it is not always clear that water rather than solid ground lies beneath.

MARGINAL IRIS AND CANDELABRA PRIMULAS ARE SUITABLE
PLANTS FOR THE EDGE OF AN INFORMAL POOL.

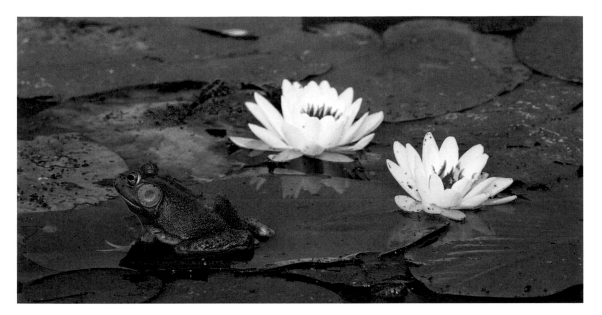

SOME SUGGESTIONS FOR WATER LILIES

Nymphaea 'Amabilis'
Candy-pink flowers with very pointed petals. Spreads to 1.2m (4ft) and needs 45–75cm (18–30in) depth of water. *Hardiness zone 5.*

Nymphaea 'Atropurpurea'
Dark crimson flowers amid reddish foliage. Spreads to 1.5m (5ft) but grows in shallow water of 30–60cm (2–3ft). *Hardiness zone 5.*

Nymphaea x *helvola*
A hybrid suitable for the tiniest of ponds. Starry, yellow flowers freely produced. Spreads only to 10–20cm (4–8in) across and will grow in a tub water feature. *Hardiness zone 4.*

Nymphaea odorata
A pure white species spreading to 1.2m (4ft) and needing water depth of 45–75cm (18–30in). *Hardiness zone 5.*

Nymphaea 'Perry's Pink'
Mauvish pink flowers, foliage bronze when young. Spreads to 1.2m (4ft) in 45–75cm (18–30in) water. *Hardiness zone 5.*

Nymphaea 'Texas Dawn'
An American cultivar with primrose flowers of great elegance. Spreads to 1.2m (4ft) in water 45–75cm (18–30in) deep. *Hardiness zone 6.*

Nymphaea 'William Falconer'
Dark red with purple-veined leaves. Spreads to 1.2m (4ft) in 45–75cm (18–30in) water. *Hardiness zone 5.*

CHOOSE WATER LILIES ACCORDING TO THEIR VIGOUR AND THE SIZE OF YOUR POOL.
LILY PADS SHADE THE WATER AND IMPROVE ITS QUALITY.

A PLACE FOR SELF-EXPRESSION

The garden is one of the few places where you can express yourself freely and creatively. It is a space to create 'the world as wanted' – even though to others that world may look messy and overgrown, bizarre, or simply in bad taste.

At Crystal Palace Park in south London there is a landscape complete with life-size model dinosaurs emerging from the undergrowth, so that you can imagine yourself back in the prehistoric era. The Georgians delighted in such ideas in the eighteenth century, creating classic landscapes with temples and ruins, and even employing hermits to inhabit rustic grottoes. The Victorians, too, conjured up worlds within worlds: at Biddulph Grange, in Staffordshire, there are gardens representing ancient Egypt and China. This is paralleled today by Sir Geoffrey Jellicoe's Moody Gardens, a vast 'garden of gardens' on the coast of the Gulf of Mexico in which every national style of garden is represented from classical times to the present. This is a large version of what many of us do on a far smaller scale – we create a patch that is our own and in a style that gives us pleasure and recreation.

AN ARMILLARY SPHERE EVOKES THE MOTION OF THE SPHERES AND THE PASSAGE OF TIME.

Using ornament in the garden

One of the quickest and easiest ways of demonstrating individuality or creating another world in your garden is through the use of ornament. What you choose will speak volumes about your interests and predilections and will perform the essential functions of all art, to surprise and to disturb as well as to please.

Ornament can range from the very traditional to minimalist, from romantic to quirky and eccentric; from a stone statue to a row of brightly painted watering cans, from a mosaic insert in paving to a weather-vane in the shape of a witch on a broomstick.

Ornament has been a traditional element in the design of a good garden since Roman times, and it has always had a wide variety of functions. On large estates, in the form of imposing sculpture, in stone, marble, lead or bronze, it expressed the power and wealth of the owner. In many domestic gardens, however, sculpted material frequently had a practical as well as a decorative purpose: for example, assisting with telling the time or covering a wellhead. But ornament can be much more; it can summon association and stir memories. A classic urn, for example, would say something about tradition and respect for the past, but might also evoke memories about where it was acquired and the person who acquired it. The way that ornament is used in the garden can also evoke different moods. Thus an old sewing machine stand or single metal chair

GARDENS CAN BE QUIRKY AND THE QUIRKINESS CAN REMAIN PERSONAL (AS OPPOSITE) OR BECOME FAMOUS LIKE DEREK JARMAN'S GARDEN AT DUNGENESS, KENT.

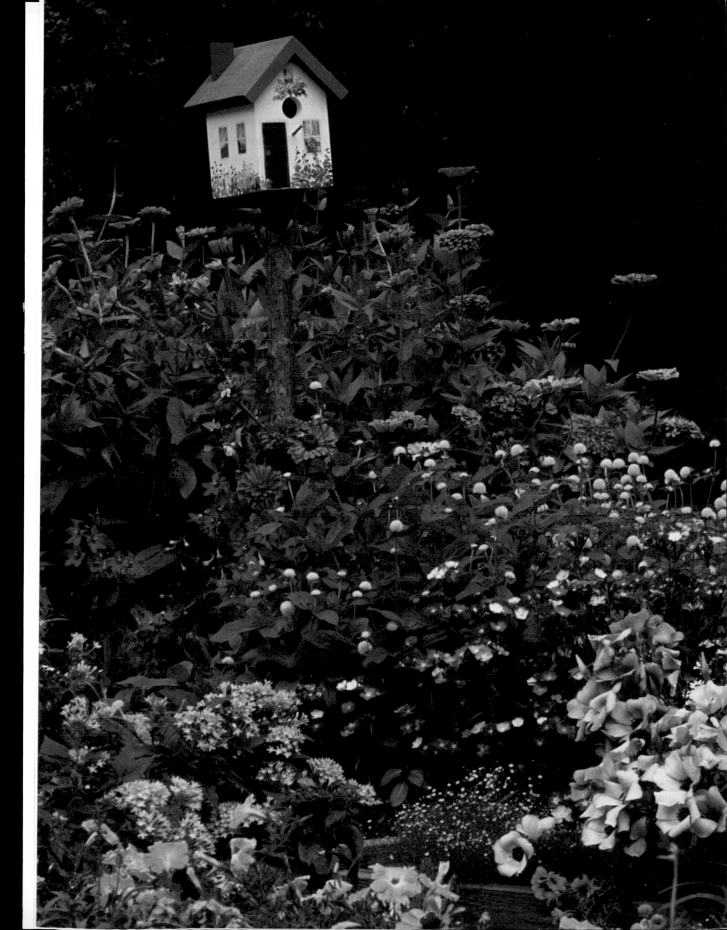

THE END OF THE DAY

'In puffs of balm the night-air blows
The perfume which the day fore-goes
And on the pure horizon far,
See, pulsing with the first-born star,
The liquid sky above the hill!
The evening comes, the fields are still.'

Matthew Arnold (1822–88)

Gardens have a particularly soothing quality at the end of the day as the plants recover from heat and revive in the cool of the evening. Sometimes you can almost see plants recover. From a slightly wilted appearance they succeed in drawing up water at a greater rate than they are losing it from their leaves. On the other hand, some plants 'go to sleep' by drooping their leaves in rest; this is a common phenomenon in shrubs belonging to the pea family, for example. The daily cycle of plants often mirrors our own moods, allowing the garden to refresh us spiritually as we recover from the stress and activity of the day and calm us before we sleep.

Providing lighting in your garden can add a magical quality to this precious time of day. It can also enable you to see the activities of nocturnal animals and the roosting of birds, all of which link you with the natural world and its processes, which have their own steady and unhurried pace. If you have a piece of sculpture or an ornament, consider lighting to bring out its full dramatic potential: floodlighting will create strong shadows and concealed uplighting can focus the eye upon an object. Pools of water can also be floodlit from above or illuminated by submerged lights (but a qualified contractor must be used for this type of installation to ensure the safe use of electrical equipment near water).

Rest is essential to the process of healing, both spiritually and physically, and is neglected at our peril. If we are deprived of sleep we suffer psychologically, and there is some evidence that we need a chance to dream, to review the past day and its conflicts and difficulties. There are many plants that can help us do just that, by enjoying their benefits in the form of herbal teas (see page 52) or using them to make a sweet-smelling pillow.

HOW TO MAKE A HERB PILLOW

Choose a pillowcase or cushion cover to suit the décor of your bedroom. Fill it with dried hop flowers, best obtained in the late autumn. Add a generous sprinkling of lavender flowers to the mixture and zip up the pillow. Place the pillow under your head to help you to sleep. The hop perfume induces sleep and the lavender is a relaxant. Refresh the mixture every few months by adding a few drops of essential oil of lavender to the mixture. Happy dreams!

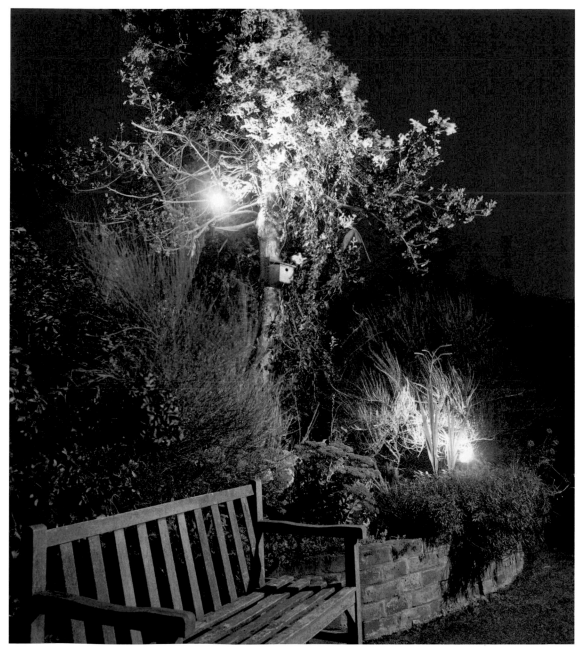

But surely the most important joy of a garden in the evening, especially on a warm summer's evening, is its sense of well-being, of containment of the human spirit and its allowance and acceptance of approaching rest: paradise found, the return to Eden.

LIGHTING HELPS US ENJOY THE SPECIAL QUALITIES OF A GARDEN IN THE EVENING
AND PROLONGS THE USE OF OUTSIDE SPACE.

AUTHOR'S ACKNOWLEDGEMENTS

Many thanks to Penny Hammond for considerable feedback and assistance; Dr Arthur Hollman for advice and technical information on double-blind tested drugs; Susyn Andrews for taxonomic assistance on lavenders; the Wellcome Galleries of the History of Medicine; Roy Genders for his work towards classification of plant perfumes; Penelope Hobhouse for her pioneering work on the history of colour; and Hilary Duckett for typing.

The table on page 51 owes much to the work of Dr Arthur Hollman of the Royal College of Physicians of London and lately Adviser to the Chelsea Physic Garden.

The table on page 125 is based on Roy Genders' *Scented Flora of the World: An Encyclopaedia* (1978).

The recipe for pot-pourri on page 133 is reprinted from *The Book of the Rose* by Michael Gibson (Macdonald, 1980).

PHOTOGRAPHIC CREDITS
ALAMY: pp.12 Andrew Butler/National Trust Photo Library, 18 Luigi Galperti/CuboImages SRL, 50 + 56 Paroli Galperti/CuboImages SRL, 59 Andrew Lawson Photography, 64 Amanda D'Arcy, 74 Peter Dean/Agripicture Images, 77 Harald Theissen/ Imagebrokers, 81 Agrophotos, 88 Paroli Galperti/ CuboImages SRL, 97 Elizabeth Whiting & Associates, 102 Gay Bumgarner, 105 Andrew Lawson Photography, 121 Angela Jordan, 139 Media Colors, 146/7 Michael Juno, 154 Gay Bumgarner, 156 Hortus, 162 Brad Mitchell, 165 Paul Shawcross/ Leslie Garland Picture Library, 167 (right) Paroli Galperti/ CuboImages SRL, 173 Gay Bumgarner, 177 Elizabeth Whiting & Associates

ALAMY/Garden Picture Library: pp. 24 Howard Rice, 42 Marie O'Hara, 47 Howard Rice, 53 A.I. Lord, 55 Suzie Gibbons, 70 Juliette Eade, 73 Jo Whitworth, 75 Christi Carter, 79 Steven Wooster, 80 Mayer/Le Scanff, 84 Eric Crichton, 87 Suzie Gibbons, 89 Lynne Brotchie, 92 Howard Rice, 93 Linda Burgess (StillLife), 98 Marie O'Hara, 99 J.S. Sira, 100 (left) Steven Wooster, 100 (right) Sunniva Harte, 103 + 114 Howard Rice, 118 (right) Mark Bolton, 122 Ron Evans, 123 Neil Holmes, 128 John Glover, 137 Andrea Jones, 148 Henk Dijkman, 149 Juliette Wade, 150 Ron Sutherland, 151 Juliette Wade, 153 + 155 Ron Sutherland, 157 Frederic Didillon, 160 Sunniva Harte, 166 Didier Willery, 168 Ron Sutherland, 172 Juliette Wade, 181 Bob Challinor

CORBIS: pp.19 The Cover Story, 37 Michael S. Yamashita, 40 Kevin Shafer, 41 Louise Gubb, 44 + 65 Michael Boys, 66 Eric Crichton, 90/91 Michael Boys, 94 Michael John, 95 Michael Boys, 106 + 107 Eric Crichton, 108 Michael Boys, 116 Eric Crichton, 118 (left) Martin B Withers/Frank Lane Agency, 127 Tania Midgely, 134 Tony Wharton/Frank Lane Picture Agency, 138 Tania Midgely, 142 Michael Boys, 152 Eric Crichton, 158 Tania Midgely, 159 Eric Crichton, 161 Tania Midgely, 164 Robert Estall, 167 (left) + 169 +170 + 179 Eric Crichton

Eden Project: pp. 21, 23, 34, 46, 48, 52, 69, 86, 110, 129, 135, 163, 174, 175

International Centre for Conservation Education: p. 39

Sue Minter: pp. 30, 113, 131, 140, 144

NASA: p. 33

Edward Parker: p. 63

USDA: p. 78

FURTHER READING
All publications are British unless otherwise noted.

CHAPTER ONE
THE HEALING ARTS
Bensky and Gamble *Chinese Herbal Materia Medica* (Eastland Press, US, 1986)

Ballick, M.J. and Cox, P.A. *Plants, People and Culture: The Science of Ethnobotany* (Scientific American Library, 1996)

Buckman, R. and Sabbagh, K. *Magic or Medicine? An Investigation into Healing* (Macmillan, 1993)

Castro, M. *The Complete Homeopathy Handbook* (Macmillan, 1990)

Chrishti, H. *The Traditional Healer* (Thorsons, 1988)

Cribb, A.B. and J.W. *Wild Medicine in Australia* (Angus and Robertson, Aust., 1992)

Culpeper, Nicholas *Culpeper's Complete Herbal* (1653) (reprint Omega, 1985)

Davis, P. *Aromatherapy, an A–Z* (C.W. Daniel, 1988)

Grieve, M.A. *A Modern Herbal* (Tiger Books, 1992)

Griggs, B. *Green Pharmacy: A History of Herbal Medicine* (Jill Norman and Hobhouse, 1981)

Hayfield, Robin *Homeopathy for Common Ailments* (Angus and Robertson, Aust., 1992)

Heyn, B. *Ayurvedic Medicine* (Thorsons, 1987)

Hollman, A. *Pharmaceutical Plants in Medicine* (Chelsea Physic Garden, 2000)

Kaptchuk, T. and Croucher, M. *The Healing Arts* (BBC Books, 1986)

Lange, D. *Europe's Medicinal and Aromatic Plants: Their Use, Trade and Conservation* (Traffic International, Cambridge, 1998)

Lange, D. and Schippman, U. *Trade Survey of Medicinal Plants in Germany* (Bundesamt für Naturschutz, Germany, 1997)

Lockie, Dr. A. *The Family Guide to Homeopathy* (Elm Tree Books, 1989)

Lovelock, James *Gaia: A New Look at Life on Earth* (OUP, 1979) and *The Ages of Gaia: A Biography of Our Living Planet* (OUP, 1988)

Lyons, A.S. and Petrucelli, R.J. *Medicine: An Illustrated History* (Abradale Press, New York, 1987)

Minter, S.A. *The Apothecaries' Garden: A History of Chelsea Physic Garden* (Sutton Publishing, 2000)

Price, Shirley *Practical Aromatherapy* (Thorsons, 1987) and *Aromatherapy for Common Ailments* (Angus and Robertson, Aust., 1992)

Stockwell, C. *Nature's Pharmacy* (Century, 1988)

CHAPTER TWO
NATURE'S PHARMACY
Baker, Harry *The Fruit Garden Displayed* (Royal Horticultural Society, 1991)

Bown, Deni *Herbal* (Pavilion Books, 2001)

Boxer, A. and Back, P. *The Herb Book* (Octopus Books, 1980)

Buczacki, S. and Harris, K. *The Collins Guide to Pests, Diseases and Disorders of Garden Plants* (Collins, 1981)

Cartwright, Lorna *A Common Sense Guide to Medicinal Plants* (Angus and Robertson, Aust., 1985)

Dudley, N. and Stickland, S. *G is for Eco Garden* (Gaia Books, 1991)

Evans, M. *A Guide to Herbal Remedies* (C.W. Daniel, 1990) and *Herbal Plants* (Studio Editions, 1991)

Holt, Geraldine *The Gourmet Garden* (Pavilion Books, 1990)

Larkom, Joy *The Salad Garden* (Windward, 1984), *The Vegetable Garden Displayed* (Royal Horticultural Society, 1992) and *Oriental Vegetables* (John Murray, 1991)

Leung, A.Y. *Encyclopaedia of Common Natural Ingredients Used in Food, Drugs and Cosmetics* (John Wiley, Chichester and New York, 1980)

Lewington, A. *Plants for People* (revised edition, Eden Project Books, 2003)

McIntyre, Anne *Herbs for Common Ailments* (Angus and Robertson, Aust., 1992)

Polunin, M. and Robbins, C. *The Natural Pharmacy* (Dorling Kindersley, 1992)

Richardson, R. *The Little Garlic Book* (Piatkus, 1982)

Swanson, Faith *Herb Garden Design* (Hanover, NH, University Press of New England, 1984)

Vaughan, J.G. and Geissler, C.A. *The New Oxford Book of Food Plants* (OUP, 1997)

Wren, R.C. *Potter's New Cyclopaedia of Botanical Drugs and Preparations* (Daniel, 1988)

CHAPTER THREE

AWAKENING THE SENSES

Archer-Wills, A. *The Water Gardener* (Frances Lincoln, 1993)

Fleet, K. *Gardening without Sight* (RNIB, 1989)

Genders, R. *Scented Flora of the World* (Robert Hale, 1994)

Hemphill, Rosemary *Cooking with Herbs and Spices* (Angus and Robertson, Aust., 1977), *Fragrance and Flavour* (Angus and Robertson, Aust., 1984) and *Herbs for all Seasons* (Angus and Robertson, Aust., 1992)

Hobhouse, Penelope *Colour in Your Garden* (Collins, 1985; Boston, Little Brown, 1985)

Houdret, J. *Pomanders, Posies and Pot-pourri* (Shire, 1988)

Jekyll, Gertrude *Colour in the Flower Garden* (Country Life, 1908)

Lacey, Stephen *Scent in Your Garden* (Angus and Robertson, Aust., 1991)

Lloyd, Christopher *Foliage Plants* (Random House, 1985)

Loewenfeld, C. and Back, P. *Herbs for Health and Cookery* (Pan Books, 1965)

Lord, T. *Encyclopaedia of Planting Combinations* (Firefly Books Ltd 2003)

Page, M. and Stearn, W.T. *Culinary Herbs* (Wisley Handbook 16, The Royal Horticultural Society, 1979)

Weiss, E.A. *Essential Oil Crops* (CAB International, 1997)

Wright, M. *The Complete Handbook of Garden Plants* (Michael Joseph, 1984)

CHAPTER FOUR

A SPIRITUAL HAVEN

Andy Goldsworthy (by Himself) (Viking, 1990)

Baines, C. *How to Make a Wildlife Garden* (Elm Tree Books, 1985)

Banks, Elizabeth *Creating Period Gardens* (Phaidon, 1991)

Bazin, Germain *Paradeisos, The Art of the Garden* (Cassell, 1990)

Hagedorn, R. *Therapeutic Horticulture* (Winslow Press, 1987)

Hunt, Peter *The Book of Garden Ornaments* (Dent, 1974)

Jellicoe, G.A. and S. *The Landscape of Man* (Thames and Hudson, 1975)

Jellicoe, Good and Lancaster *The Oxford Companion to Gardens* (Oxford University Press, 1991)

Laird, M. *The Formal Garden* (Thames and Hudson, 1992)

Phillips, R. and Rix, M. *Conservatory and Indoor Plants Vols 1 & 2* (Macmillan, 1997)

Please, P. (ed.) *Able to Garden: A Practical Guide for Disabled and Elderly Gardeners* (Batsford 1990)

Smit, T. *Eden* (Bantam Press, 2001)

Stoneham, J.A. and Thoday, P.R. *Landscape Design for Elderly and Disabled People* (Antique Collectors Club, Garden Art Press, Woodbridge, Suffolk, 1994)

Taylor, G. and Cooper, G. *Gardens of Obsession* (Cassell, 2000)

Ten Kate, K. and Laird, S.A. *The Commercial Use of Biodiversity* (Earthscan, 1999)

Verey, R. *Garden Plans* (Frances Lincoln, 1993)

USEFUL ADDRESSES AND WEBSITES

The Dr Edward Bach Centre (Bach Flower
Remedies), Mount Vernon, Sotwell, Wallingford,
Oxon OX10 0PZ

British Herbal Medicine Association, P.O. Box 304,
Bournemouth, Dorset BH7 6JZ
www.ex.ac.uk/phytonet/bhma.html

Chelsea Physic Garden, 66 Royal Hospital Road,
London SW3 4HS
www.chelseaphysicgarden.co.uk

Henry Doubleday Research Association (for
information on organic gardening), Ryton Gardens,
Ryton-on-Dunsmore, Coventry CV8 3LG

Gardening for Disabled Trust, Church Cottage,
Headcorn, Kent TN27 9NP

The Herb Society, Sulgrave Manor, Sulgrave,
Banbury, Oxon OX17 2SD
www.herbsociety.co.uk

Horticultural Trades Association, Horticulture
House, 19 High Street, Theale RG7 5AH
www.the-hta.com

Medicines Control Agency
(herbal medicine safety website)
www.mca.gov.uk/aboutagency/regframework/csm/
csmhome.htm

National Institute of Medical Herbalists,
56 Longbrook Street, Exeter, Devon EX4 6AH
www.nimh.org.uk

Plants for People
www.plantsforpeople.org
Contact www.the-hta.org.uk – go to plantforlife.info

Royal Blind Society, Torwood, Ashley Lane, Winsley,
Bradford on Avon BA15 2HR

Royal National Institute for the Blind, 105 Judd
Street, London WC1H 9NE
www.rnib.org.uk

Royal Society for the Protection of Birds (RSPB),
The Lodge, Sandy, Bedfordshire SG19 2DL
www.rspb.org.uk

The Sensory Trust, Watering Lane Nursery,
Pentewan, St Austell, Cornwall PL26 6BE
www.sensorytrust.org.uk

Soil Association (for information on organic
gardening), 40–56 Victoria Street, Bristol BS1 6BY
www.soilassociation.org

Stannah Stairlifts (garden stairlifts), Watt Close,
East Parkway, Andover, Hants SP10 3SD
www.stannah.co.uk/stairlifts

Thrive, The Geoffrey Udall Centre, Beech Hill,
Reading RG7 2AT
www.thrive.org.uk

CONTROVERSIES

Chinese Medicinal Plant Authentication Centre
www.rbgkew.org.uk

Fairtrade Foundation
www.fairtrade.org.uk

Medicinal Plant Specialist Group of IUCN Species
Survival Commission
www.mpsg.org

Rainforest Alliance
www.rainforest-alliance.org

Transforming Violence
www.transformingviolence.org

LIST OF SUPPLIERS

HERBS – SEEDS AND PLANTS

Suttons Seeds, Torbay, England – *Seeds*.
www.suttons-seeds.co.uk

Norfolk Lavender Ltd, Caley Mill, Heacham,
Norfolk PE31 7JE – *Plants*
www.norfolklavender.co.uk

ORGANICALLY GROWN HERBS, SEEDS AND PRODUCTS

Jekka's Herb Farm, Rose Cottage, Shellards Lane,
  Alveston, Bristol BS35 3SY
  www.jekkasherbfarm.com
Suffolk Herbs, Monk's Farm, Kelvedon, Colchester,
  Essex CO5 9PG
  www.suffolkherbs.com
The Organic Herb Trading Company, Milverton,
  Somerset TA4 1NF
  www.organicherbtrading.com

HERBS – PRODUCTS

G. Baldwin & Co. 171–173 Walworth Road,
  London SE17 1RW
  www.baldwins.co.uk
Potters (Herbal Supplies) Ltd, Leyland Mill Lane,
  Wigan, WN1 2SB
  www.pottersherbals.co.uk

ORGANIC CONTROL OF PESTS

Koppert (UK) Ltd, Homefield Road, Haverhill,
  Suffolk CB9 8QP
  www.koppert.nl

WATER GARDENING

Alnwick Garden, Northumberland
  www.alnwickgarden.com
  (see index on homepage)
Stapeley Water Gardens Ltd, Stapeley, Nantwich,
  Cheshire CW5 7LH
  www.stapeleywatergardens.com
Maydencroft Aquatic Nurseries, Maydencroft Lane,
  Gosmore, Hitchin, Herts SG4 7QD
  www.maydencroftaquatics.com

AROMATHERAPY OILS AND SUPPLIERS

Bay House Aromatics, 88 St Georges Road,
  Brighton BN2 1EE
  www.bayhousearomatics.co.uk

Culpeper Ltd, 21 Bruton Street, London W1J 6QD
  (and countrywide)
  www.culpeper.co.uk

PERIOD GARDEN FURNITURE, TROMPE L'OEIL AND SCULPTURE

Andrew Crace Designs, 51 Bourne Lane,
  Much Hadham, Herts SG10 6ER
  www.andrewcrace.com
The Landscape Ornament Company,
  www.landscapeornament.com

TERRACOTTA POTS

Creta Cotta, Jubilee Cottage, Penrhos, Raglan,
  Monmouthshire NP15 2LE
  www.cretacotta.co.uk
Whichford Pottery, Whichford, Shipton-on-Stour,
  Warwickshire CV36 5PG
  www.whichfordpottery.com

UNUSUAL AND TENDER PLANTS

Architectural Plants, Nuthurst, Horsham,
  West Sussex RH13 6LH
  www.architecturalplants.com
Chiltern Seeds, Bortree Stile, Ulverston,
  Cumbria LA12 7PB
  www.chilternseeds.co.uk
Hopley's Plants Ltd, High Street, Much Hadham,
  Herts SG10 6BU
  www.hopleys.co.uk

Refer also to nurseries listed in:
  Tony Lord (ed.) *RHS Plant Finder,* published yearly
  by the Royal Horticultural Society
  www.rhs.org.uk/publications/index.asp

WILDFLOWERS – SEEDS AND PLANTS

Landlife Wild Flowers Ltd, National Wildflower
  Centre, Court Hey Park, Liverpool L16 3NA
  www.wildflower.org.uk

INDEX

Page numbers in italics refer to illustrations or text within boxes